The Do What You Love Diet

Finally, Finally, Finally Feel Good in Your Own Skin

by

Jen Ward
Self-Proclaimed "Unfitness Expert"

Jen Ward RM, LMT

Copyright 2016 by Jen Ward

All Rights Reserved. No part of this publication may be reproduced in any form or by any means, including scanning, photocopying, or otherwise without prior written permission of the copyright holder.

ISBN-13: 978-1537020372

ISBN-10: 1537020374

2016-: ORIGINAL VERSION 001

2016 NOVEMBER: VERSION 002

Table of Contents:

Introduction 2

Weekly Taps and Contemplations 5

Testimonials 185

About the Author 188

Jen's Books 191

Introduction

I am not a fitness expert. I am an unfitness expert. I think the problem with some fitness experts is that they don't always know exactly what the person they are assisting is experiencing. One can only have true compassion for an experience they have endured. I truly believe that I have the understanding and compassion for every experience imaginable with unfitness.

I have experienced them all. In fact, my life has been one big field study in understanding how anyone who deals with weight issues and self-esteem fails to cope. Anyone who says simply to eat less and exercise more does not know the gray area of frustration and self-loathing that goes into the inability to do just that. Just keep your mouth closed, right? No. It is not that easy. There are layer upon layer of reasons why people don't just lose weight. Sure, guilt and shame are a part of that, but what is causing the shame goes undetected. Until now. The exercises and tapping series that are provided in this book strip off layers of primal, genetic and emotional issues in regard to overeating. For example, the binge is sometimes the primal urge to hunt and gather. That was such a simpler time in our development that we attempt to conjure it back up by collecting the food, which may create more satisfaction than eating it. Or, eating at large gatherings is so pleasant because in treacherous times, eating with a large group literally signified peace. Because a large meal wouldn't be happening if there was any hint of danger.

For some people, being thin triggers past lives when they had starved to death. On some level, eating is literally a matter of life and death. Mindless eating is, many times, passing the food through their physical body to a version of themselves that is suffering. When dieticians tell you to practice mindful eating, this is the process they are asking you to interrupt. It does work. It also works to pour love and nurturing into every aspect of you on every level. When you do this, the gorging no longer is necessary to try to save yourself. Your new state of self-love permeates every aspect of you. The eating frenzy and the cycle of shame is no longer necessary.

Sometimes, we stay in a bigger body to keep people away from us. In some lifetimes, we may have been used, passed around or even sacrificed for our beauty. In those instances, the most nurturing thing to do is to ensure that no one be attracted to you in any way. Carbon, which is what fat is composed of, has a repelling quality to its nature. It is the perfect armor to prevent anyone from receiving the wrong attention. It is a form of hiding in plain sight, which so many of you have experienced. No, you are not un-loveable. You are experiencing the impersonal nature of being engulfed in the repelling nature of carbon.

This book addresses all the above issues and more. It creates such a deep understanding of our own process in regard to food and our physicality that self-compassion and care are inevitable. The tapping sequences work deeper than any other self-monitoring system works, like affirmations or psyching one's self out in an attempt to bypass the mind's permission. The brain has been monitoring every attempt to change your current health status. It is satisfied with you now or else you would be different. This book changes the mindset so that the physicality follows instead of trying to change the physicality, by working against the mindsets already in play.

So I am not a fitness expert. I have not even solved this issue for myself. Perhaps I am still doing research. But so many people around me, who are using my techniques, have reached their ideal weight and vigor without a fraction of the angst they have wasted on the pursuit thus far. In fact, reaching an ideal fitness goal was a byproduct of working on a more empowered emotional and mental state. Reaching a long-ago forgotten fitness goal became a natural process of releasing all the layers of issues that the exercises I provide here eliminate.

This is my intention for every one of you reading this book and for the whole world. We have all been at the mercy of an issue that does not empower us. It is time for you to meet the depth of your awesomeness. You will appreciate yourself at a deeper level and change in such a profound way through using the exercises in this book. Be sure to do them all. Because the ones that the mind tells you don't pertain to you, this same mind "dysregulated" your physicality in the first place.

WEEK 1

Why affirmations may not work:

When one does an affirmation, it is meant to program the mind for success. The problem is that the mind has a long memory and a strong opinion. For every positive affirmation one tries to do, the mind has access to many examples of how that is not true and refutes it. The mind refuting it can ingrain behavior even more.

For instance, if someone wants to lose weight, they may say an affirmation like, "I am happy at my perfect weight." The mind immediately starts thinking about all the diets that have failed, how unhappy it is to be overweight and maybe even could pull up memories of when the person was at that ideal weight and unhappy. It seems more futile than before that affirmation.

I help clients overcome that hurdle by giving them affirmations that the mind cannot refute or by using EFT (emotional freedom technique) taps that the mind cannot negate as easily. EFT taps are very effective in sidestepping the conscious mind and making energetic shifts. The affirmations deal with the body as a whole; the mind can't refute the mechanical workings of the body. Also, I consider the whole self to be a sound frequency or a light emanation. The mind does not have the ability to interfere with shifts because it is used to dealing in a concrete concept of the self.

Say each statement three times out loud while CONTINUOUSLY tapping on the top of your head at the crown chakra, and say it a fourth time while tapping on your chest at the heart chakra. Say each word deliberately. They are not just words but a vibration that you are initiating to shift energy. Pause after each word. Say it in a commanding but even tone, not as a question. Forgo saying it in a singsong tone or with bravado. Say them all.

Here is how I would change affirmations to EFT taps to be more effective and beneficial.

Change the affirmation *I am happy* to the EFT taps below:

"*I remove all sadness from my sound frequency; in all moments,*" and
"*I release resonating with being sad; in all moments.*"

Change the affirmation *I am my ideal weight* to the EFT taps:

"*I remove all excess from every cell in my body; in all moments*" and
"*I remove all fat from my sound frequency; in all moments*" and
"*I release resonating with being fat; in all moments*"

It may seem subtle but the mind cannot prevent change when the affirmations aren't referring to the whole or collective of what the mind has sovereign over. Success is no longer hit or miss or for the lucky few, but for all.

~ ~ ~ ~ ~

Breaking News: The Diet No More Tap

When people know that they have to lose weight, they carry around a foreboding thought of self-loathing or gloom about it. They are eating shame and remorse at every meal. It is that thought that is programming the body to gain weight. The mind registers our every thought and manifests them as required. It does not pick and choose. It does not discern. Every thought is intricately registered and processed as our new reality.

When people are successful in anything, it is because their mind is being fed a continuous stream of healthy thoughts that they are manifesting. Those who are not successful are grappling with the dance between positive suggestions to the mind and the subliminal sabotaging thoughts that play so heavily into our reality.

This is why affirmations may work for some. But for so many, while they are saying a positive statement, their mind is in overdrive pointing out all the times that they have failed. The mind can actually conjure up accounts of all the varying times that one has failed. The mind is the equivalent of having a nagging spouse with perfect recall and no filter. This is what we deal with when we are trying to achieve something new for ourselves. This is how we are our own worst enemy.

We have all known this self-sabotaging feature and have just succumbed to its process. It takes so much energy to combat this internal process that so many of us have given up hope and are resolved to complacency. But it is not necessary. The tapping exercises that I provide counter the self-sabotaging byproduct of a discerning mind.

By tapping a positive statement into the head, you are telling the conscious mind to override all other information and program the body with this new information. If the body were a news organization, it would be like interrupting the regular programming to bring breaking news about an important current event.

Tapping on the head while stating a positive affirmation interrupts the regular scheduled program of negativity that is so easily programmed into the body. Tapping on the chest while continuing to say the same positive affirmation sets this information as highest priority for the body always. Saying, "in all moments," is a distinct must of the protocol that I have developed. It reassures that the body does not revert to negative programming in an attempt to shift back into complacency.

Once the positive programming is done this way, it sets precedence for the whole system. That is why the taps I post are life changing and perhaps world changing if enough people would interrupt their complacency programming to do them.

For people who want to lose weight, all they do is focus on how bad they feel about themselves for being overweight. It is a constant barrage of negative thoughts every time they eat, look in the mirror, put on clothes, groom, see other people, shop, etc. In fact, the only time they may have success in quieting the mind is when they engage in mind numbing activities like video games or watching TV. But they will only succeed in quieting the conscious thoughts, not the onslaught of subliminal thoughts or the programming process of all the negative thoughts that they already put into play.

~ ~ ~ ~ ~

Here is the life altering solution. Simply say this statement three times while tapping on your head and say it a fourth time while tapping on your chest. **(Be sure to always pause before saying "in all moments." The semicolon is there to remind you to pause.)**

"I am happy and excited to be experiencing a healthy, fit and trim body; in all moments."

You only have to say each tapping exercise once for it to override all the negative damage of the programming that has already been done. But it if you want a daily tap to do to reassure yourself, say the above tap daily or say your ideal age and weight three times as say you continuously tap on the top of your head and a forth time as you tap on your chest

It may not seem earth shaking at first, but what you may find is that you start to notice healthy thoughts about yourself slipping into your conscious mind.

Often people start to feel hope about losing weight. They start making slightly better food choices. They start gaining momentum in the process, and they turn the whole dynamic of dieting into a life-altering, exciting current and ongoing event.

This is also an effective technique for those who are aging and live in a society that focuses so much of attention on aging, disease and death. Here is a daily tap for anyone who feels the effect of negative programming in any one of those areas.

"I enjoy a perpetual state of Joy, health and vigor at all ages; in all moments."

There is a reason that this information is being given to you now and you are able to receive it. The world is moving towards a state of regeneration and a state of contentment that it has never realized before. Consciousness is not a static state. It is always changing. Here is to being a part of the process of playing catch up to the incredible higher consciousness that we are all immersed in. It is already here. We, in our human consciousness, are merely dipping our toe in gradually. How gradually is up to each individual. But at a point, we will all dive in. Higher consciousness is an exhilarating wonderment. Come on in. The water is fine.

WEEK 2

You Deserve Wellness

When people have an issue, they many times think in the worse case scenario. Even when deciding whether they are coming down with a flu or something, they have to ruminate over the signs before they validate themselves by telling others they are sick.

Then they feel the need to defend those issues. They don't want to sound ridiculous, so they build up a case for being sick. They are, in a sense, coming to agreement with the illness. Then they identify with it by defending their need to nurture themselves by having it.

Being sick is a chance to opt out for a bit. It is an excuse to stay home, relinquish the diet, forgo the work load, spoil oneself, relax, take a break, feel important, be the center of attention, ask for help, surrender to life, allow others to help and change priorities. Because people are used to invalidating themselves otherwise, being sick is their chance to get fulfillment, at first.

But then the novelty rubs off and the patient feels they have to return to 'the grind" or up the anti on their illness. It is sad to think how many people up the anti. It is one of the main reasons dis-ease is so prevalent in society.

Here is a better way: take a day off, go off the diet once in awhile, spoil yourself, leave work at the office, be the center of attention, accept help, ask for help, change priorities, have fun, return to joy, return to ease. Create it! Demand it! Revel in it. What the human can endure is limited, but what the human spirit can tap into is infinite.

~ ~ ~ ~ ~

Here are some EFT taps to help:

(Say each statement three times while tapping on your head and say it a forth time while tapping on your chest)

"I release validating myself through illness; in all moments."
"I release using illness to relate to others; in all moments." (this may happen in genetic diseases)
"I release my genetic propensity for disease; in all moments."
"I release carrying illness in my DNA; in all moments."
"I release using illness to feel special; in all moments."
"I release using illness as a common ground; in all moments."
"I release being in agreement with illness; in all moments."
"I remove being cursed with illness; in all moments."

~ ~ ~ ~ ~ ~

"I dissolve all karmic ties with illness; in all moments."

"I remove all the pain, burden and limitations that illness has put on me; in all moments."
"I take back all the joy, love, abundance and freedom that illness has taken from me; in all moments."
"I release resonating with illness; in all moments."
"I release all illness from my sound frequency; in all moments."
"I shift my paradigm from illness to joy, love, abundance and freedom; in all moments."

Let's return to Joy, Love, Abundance and Freedom. Those are birthrights worth striving for and what every loving parent wishes for their baby. You deserve a wonderful existence.

WEEK 3

A New Approach to Healthy Living: The Thought Diet

I have a great plan to help people lose weight, avoid bouts of depression, to help them in relationships and with their overall wellbeing. Rather than being concerned with all the outer stimuli in your environment, how about if you paid total attention to how you process it?

For instance, every time you take a bite of food, instead of telling yourself something negative as you eat it, why not tell yourself you are doing something good for yourself? Why eat guilt every time you eat a couple extra calories? It isn't going to help you in any stretch of the imagination to tell yourself how undisciplined you are for enjoying what you are enjoying.

Abstain from telling yourself that "you are going to pay for this later," or that you are "being bad," or that "you really shouldn't." Why not turn every situation around so it is a benefit to yourself and others who are in close proximity and are learning by your example? Why not tell yourself that this is exactly what you need in the moment and that you are enjoying the experience? If your body did not crave or want it on some level, you wouldn't be eating it anyway. Even if it feels like you are being self-indulgent, tell yourself that you deserve it. You do.

Forego berating yourself over minute issues. Make everything you do in your day a positive. Be an example to others in this way and you will see how much easier it is to stay positive overall.

~ ~ ~ ~ ~

Another way we indulge is in world affairs. It seems that there is a mass negative outlook of the world. That is because so many are watching the news and filtering negativity into their world and identifying with it. The world is a constant. Human nature hasn't changed. There have always been crises in the world. There have always been natural and man-made disasters in the world. Some people are learning their spiritual lessons by breaking man-made laws. That is a process of learning that they need. We don't need to involve ourselves in everyone else's experiences.

We manifest our view of the world through our understanding of it. If all we focus on are crimes and deficiencies, we will feel like a victim and feel a lack of abundance. Our natural state is one of Love, Beauty, Joy, and Abundance. The less we bring the negative experiences of others willingly into our world, the more we can enjoy our natural state. Where years ago it was a given to experience the innocence of these things, now it has become something that we need to exercise. We are becoming more aware of our own abilities to stay in a beautiful space as opposed to inflict negativity on ourselves and on those around us.

When we indulge in bouts of negativity and feeling sorry for ourselves, it is an emotional binge. It is as destructive on the psyche as indulging in a bottomless hot fudge sundae would be. One choice brings discomfort to the physical body; the other one brings dis-ease to the emotional body. Both are indulgences at their best. Sometimes our body needs a little sympathy but always in moderation, just like anything else. So instead of going through the day berating yourself and others, turn the day around with your own positive spin on the day.

Find something positive in every situation. If people are complaining about the weather, respond with a positive quip: "I bet the plants are loving the rain."

Pay attention to your thoughts through the day. Catch yourself saying anything negative and stop yourself.

~ ~ ~ ~ ~

Negative comments are so subtle sometimes we don't realize we are doing it. Ask those close to you to point out when you are saying something negative, just so you can see your own pattern and then disrupt it.

If you are eating something that you think you shouldn't, realize that you need it on some level and give yourself permission to enjoy it. That may even stop you from needing it again so soon.

Remember that you want, and sometimes desperately need, to be reassured or validated. But don't depend on others to do this for you. Do it for yourself.

Understand that everybody struggles with these issues of being human. We are not special in the fact that we are hard on ourselves. Remove the belief that you alone are having a hard time just being happy daily. By realizing others' struggle, it removes the belief that you are isolated. It also may assist in stepping up to the plate and being a positive example to others.

Realize that others are bombarded by negative stimuli. When you complain or are discouraged, they may have nothing left to give to you to assist you in feeling better. It is up to you to change your mood around for yourself and for those around you. This is spiritual maturity.

Others are not thinking about you in a negative way. If they have slighted you or hurt your feelings, they may not even realize it. You are the only one carrying it around most times. So literally drop it and let it go.

You want to change the dynamics of a situation? Shock people by taking the high ground. It will get their attention and can remove a cloud of dissent. It may just feel so good you can get in the habit of taking the high ground and be someone who stands out as a positive role model.

Be grateful. In any and every situation, be grateful. You are laden with such gifts! Please recognize them. In your ability to be grateful, you perpetuate all of the innate gifts in yourself: Beauty, Love, Freedom, Joy and Peace. And when you perpetuate them in yourself, you perpetuate them in others as well.

If you want world peace, find inner peace and bring it to others one person at a time. This is how a single match can light all the candles in a cathedral, and how your spiritual light can uplift the masses.

WEEK 4

Reasons we hold extra weight

There are many reasons why people hold extra weight on their body. In past lives, many of us have starved to death. The relationship with food is so complex. But aside from food issues, people use weight as a means to isolate themselves from the pain of interacting with others.

If someone has been devastated at the hands of others, they may use layers of fat to literally insulate themselves. Since this isn't done on a conscious level, overweight people can obsess over that extra weight. The extra weight can be a direct correlation to the pain they carry from a past life. They are indirectly obsessing over the pain that they are carrying around.

To lose the layers of fat, we may have to let go of the pain that we are storing. The physical weight is reflective of the emotional heaviness. It may be much more effective to work from the inside first.

~ ~ ~ ~ ~

(Say each statement three times while taping on your head, and say it a fourth time while tapping on your chest.)

"I release storing emotional issues in my physical body; in all moments."
"I release using my body for emotional storage; in all moments."
"I release declaring myself fat; in all moments."
"I release eating shame; in all moments."
"I release protecting myself in fat; in all moments."
"I release insulating myself from pain; in all moments."
"I recant all vows and agreements between myself and fat; in all moments."
"I remove all curses and blessings between myself and fat; in all moments."
"I dissolve all karmic ties between myself and fat; in all moments."

~ ~ ~ ~ ~

"I remove all the pain, burden and limitations that fat has put on me; in all moments."
"I take back all the Joy, Love, Abundance, Freedom, and Wholeness that fat has taken from me; in all moments."
"I release resonating with fat; in all moments."
"I remove all fat from my Sound frequency; in all moments."
"I remove all fat from my Light body; in all moments."
"I shift my paradigm from fat to Joy, Love, Abundance, Freedom, Health, and Wholeness; in all moments."

We can use positive affirmation until we are blue in the face. But sometimes, the mind will refute everything positive that we try to manifest for ourselves. It will remind us of how many times we have failed. This is a great technique in sneaking past the mind and making an energetic shift without asking the mind to be on board. The mind does not know how to refute removing fat from the sound frequency. These taps bypass the mind.

WEEK 5

Gain Awareness

Separate yourself from the experience that you are having. For example, when you are outside, the cold is striking your body, but you are not cold. Differentiate between yourself and the experience. Don't say, "I'm cold." Don't make yourself that easily swayed.

If you can separate yourself in this way, then you can also prevent yourself from getting lost in identifying with other negative things. You will stop telling yourself:

> I'm starving
> I'm fat
> I'm poor
> I'm ugly.

None of these are true statements. These statements enslave you to an exterior situation that is irrelevant to whom you are.

~ ~ ~ ~ ~

Thoughts

Thoughts and words actually have a weight to them. That is why positive words are so light and negative words are so heavy.

Technique:

Pay attention to the words that you use and the thoughts that you tell yourself. If you are feeling tired or depressed, change the words that you tell yourself. You don't have to believe them at first. In fact, the heaviness of some of the words you have been using will make it difficult for you to resonate with the positive ones you are replacing them with.

This is just a process of faith. Once you feel a shift in yourself or a more lightness of being, it will be enjoyable to consciously choose to elevate yourself.

~ ~ ~ ~ ~

Action follows thought. That is why visualizations work.

Here is a fun visualization to augment your weight loss efforts.

Visualize your body as an airport. Think of all the fat cells as travelers ready to get on a plane and fly away. Visualize them with their baggage (toxins) and you handing them all their tickets. Say goodbye graciously to them and thank them for their service. Watch all the fat cells get on their planes and create a mass exodus from your body. Watch them fly away. See the airport cleared out with clean passageways.

By using a visualization that is removed from your actual body, it alleviates the negative self-talk, feelings and beliefs. Because of its lack of association with the actual body, it prevents self-sabotage.

WEEK 6

Positive Reprogramming

We create space in this world for the things we want to manifest by what we give our attention to. That is why I don't understand why so many people talk about problems. If people don't want problems, why do they give so much life to them? Hasn't everyone had the experience by now of talking about problems and as they talk about them, they can feel more and more animation and life behind them? Why don't they stop doing this?

Opposite technique: Whatever you seem to struggle with, talk about and embellish the opposite. It can be "tongue in cheek" at first until it feels comfortable. If someone is struggling with weight issues, they would talk about what a problem it is to be so thin. Get a feeling for what that self-talk feels like or say it to another. It will bring a totally different feeling into the body. Bring a spouse or a good friend into the game and talk about any issues in opposite terms.

Use opposite terms to talk about things. Have whole conversations in opposite. It is a way to change a setting that is stuck on talking about problems. It is a great way to change self-talk. This is a great way to teach children how to be positive. They will even talk about things that they wouldn't open up about because it is fun and easy to do it in opposite terms.

Instead of hearing, "I am ugly, and all the boys hate me," a child may be able to open up and say, "I am so beautiful that all the boys love me too much" Isn't this how you would rather your child talk about themselves? Isn't it a way that you deserve to feel about yourself. It is a small discipline to put in place to really change one's quality of life.

~ ~ ~ ~ ~

Protection and a Big Body

Many people who are in a big body are using it as a form of protection. Their body is doing exactly what it needs to do to help them feel safe. Instead of appreciating this, they curse it, and this adds more disease on top of the original trauma. Then they punish it by starving it and overworking it.

Maybe a better way to deal with it is to send soothing thoughts to the body and nurture it. Send it gratitude and love. When you are kind to yourself, your self will be more willing to hone you into what the real issue is that is going on. Just like with anything else, kindness goes further when dealing with yourself.

~ ~ ~ ~ ~

Sympathy and fat have similar vibratory rates.

It is important that people realize that the feelings that we harbor in our body of anger, frustration, and shame are not merely a blanket of unworthiness. They are a rich array of experiences that need to be unwoven from our tapestry as intricately as they were woven in. There are two ways to do this: 1) either tedious, diligent, relentless effort, or 2) spontaneous awareness. I prefer to help people free themselves using the latter.

WEEK 7

Perspective

Your worst day...may be a day in the park to someone else.
Your worst meal...may be a banquet to someone else.
Your worst living conditions...may be a palace to someone else.
Your deepest disappointment...may be a dream come true to someone else.
Your worst date...may be the love of their life to someone else.
Your haziest stupor...may be a moment of clarity to someone else.
Your throw away attempt...may be the highest accomplishment to someone else.
Your failing body...may be renewed health to someone else.
Your fat pants...may be skinny pants to someone else.
Your bad luck...could be catching a break to someone else.
Your lack of gratitude...may be an insult to 90% of the planet.

~ ~ ~ ~ ~

Technique for Self Acceptance

Fat in the body is made of a string of carbon molecules. Did you know that carbon has the energetic component of repulsions? Its purpose is to keep others away. To be repulsed when looking at yourself may be no more than you merely identifying with the atoms. That is their job. That is not yours. Your job is to love and empower yourself.

When you look in the mirror, imagine that it is a hundred years ago when weight on the body was considered attractive. Shift your vantage point. When you can shift your vantage point, it will be easier to accept yourself. When you accept yourself, it will be easier to be present with yourself instead of seeing yourself from the emotional vantage point of the cells which is a primal emotion and not rational.

When you are present with yourself, you are empowered. Being empowered is no small victory. To be empowered is to be proud of yourself. So when you look in the mirror, learn to be proud of yourself for all that you are. If you could see the whole journey that you have endured, you would be much kinder to yourself. And in turn, you will be much kinder to others as well.

Live in the perpetual state of a smile.

~ ~ ~ ~ ~

Enthused and Happy!
Technique: Pay attention to the things that you tell yourself and consciously turn them around. If you are always saying in your mind (or even to other people)

that you are tired, change that to saying that you are enthused and happy.

Your mind is listening to everything that you say to know how to respond. How many people tell themselves that they are fat and unattractive? They even convince themselves and others that it is hopeless. Your mind is trying to help you by creating the you that you say you are. It doesn't realize that this is not your desired state. The mind deals in absolutes.

People convince themselves that it is their past experiences that determine their present condition, but it is actually the thought process that preceded each past experience that creates the condition that follows.

Say this statement three times while tapping on the head and a fourth time tapping on the chest:

"I shift my paradigm from victim-hood to living with powerful intention; in all moments."

WEEK 8

Our Words

Instead of blowing up and getting angry, speak your truth when it comes through, in gentle, steady increments.

Dogs don't hear negatives. If you say "no bark," they only hear the word bark and continue to bark to please you.

It is the same way with our own mind. If one says, "I don't want to be fat," the mind basically hears, "I want to be fat and will continue to serve you as it has."

Technique: Frame everything that you want to accomplish with strong positive words. It makes it even more positive to put the statement in the moment.

Instead of saying, "I don't want to be broke all the time," change it to, "I AM so rich!" It doesn't even matter if you are saying it tongue in cheek. In fact, you can make it a game with the family.

If your daughter wants to express that she is feeling unattractive, make her say it to you in the opposite, "I am so beautiful." If your boys are feeling lazy, tell them they have to tell you in the opposite, "I am feeling so peppy today." See how this internal dialogue helps the general dynamics of the family.

Also, when we are discouraged about world events, we talk about them and add more grief to the world. If someone says something positive, we label them as being out of touch. Maybe they are just using this technique. I know I am.

~ ~ ~ ~ ~

Beauty

Who we are in the physical realm is such a small component of who we really are. It is literally the tip of our iceberg. To focus so much of our attention on our physical form is a distraction from our true nature and our own truth. For us to be deceived into focusing so much attention on our body is an intentional form of distraction. It keeps us enslaved in denial of our true dynamic self. It is a lie. It is the perfect prison because we, ourselves, keep ourselves contained.

All the energy focused on our weight, features, wardrobe, hair texture, and all the accessories that that entails, is us buying into the lie. The lie is that we need to do anything outwardly to enhance our own beauty. Beauty is our innate nature.

Beauty is love, honor, kindness, integrity and truth. To be those things is to enhance that inner beauty that is unmatched by any synthetic process.

~ ~ ~ ~ ~

Technique to Loosen Your Spine

In contemplation, visualize your spine being suspended in air. Get a sense of the weight of the body elongating it with the help of gravity. Feel the vertebrae stretch apart as the weight of the body helps each little bone separate slightly from the one on top of it and below it. Visualize the thickness and space between each bone adjust to be even and the same consistency.

Visualize a firm, even grip pulling on the neck at the same time and elongating all the bones of the neck. Focus only on the elongation process and not the issues that have drawn too much of your attention.

Feel tension literally drip away. Feel all inconsistencies adjust themselves. It is as if the tissue between the bones were like tubes that were pinched and they are now readjusting themselves.

Get a sense of your whole physical body shifting, adjusting and stretching out as you do this.

WEEK 9

Reverse the Aging Process: Technique to Rejuvenate Your Endocrine System

In contemplation, pinpoint a certain time in a younger version of you when you can remember being present, aware, grateful and productive. Look at that version of you, and get a sense of remembering what it was like to be that you. In a very focused way, overlay that version of you onto you in the present. Overlay it on you, totally focused on that version of you, and allow it to sink into you.

Careful. DO NOT DO THIS IN THE OPPOSITE. Do not overlay yourself on top of the younger version of you. There may be a natural tendency to do that. But do not visit the present you into the past for this particular technique. Bring that version of you into the present.

When you have the younger version of you overlaid on top of you, visualize securing it to you in some way. Either clip it around the edges or glue it on top or just hold it in place. See it bulky on top of you, but hold tight to the younger version of you. You can even perceive the present you moving around underneath trying to break through. Allow the younger you to prevail.

Hold the younger version over the present version of you until there is no more struggle. Hold down until all the thicknesses are smoothed out and all the lumps are gone. Allow the present you to disintegrate. Be only aware of the younger you in it's place.

Shift your attention back into the present and look out of your body through the new set of younger eyes. Feel a sense of youth and empowerment. Forgo talking or focusing on anything that the old you would have focused or talked about. Retrain your dialogue to match the younger you.

~ ~ ~ ~ ~

Primal Gratitude

Go outside without a jacket in the cold weather. Go out in bare arms and legs. Not for too long, but long enough for the elements to register through the body. As you are doing this, all these primal memories of being deficient, starving and cold will stir up under the surface. You won't remember them, but your body will. It is enough of a reminder of what you have endured to get to this moment that it will trigger a very deep and profound gratitude.

You may not even realize that this whole dynamic is playing out. But it may induce a deep sense of contentment through your whole beingness when coming in from the cold. It may even be effective in creating a deep and lasting sense of gratitude in your whole self. It is like collapsing all time between a past trauma and now, and embracing an incredible shift of abundance and freedom.

~ ~ ~ ~ ~

Problems are stagnant energy like a cloud. They have weight and mass in the body. You can use all kinds of visualizations to dry it up, release it, unzip your body and just let it go. It wants to release. It is like steam in a kettle. Its last resort to get out is through thoughts and talking.

But a lot of that is transferring it to another person. When you release it through visualizations and open your body and let go, it dissipates immediately. Gone. No giving it away, no passing it on, no suffering in silence. Gone.

You can also do the taps on my page. They shift the energy drastically. You may discover yawning and breathing deep. It is evidence of the shift.

WEEK 10

Untangling the Psyche

During sessions, unusual connections are discovered with experiences that don't represent the standard definition. The psyche tangles reactions to something pleasant because of an overwhelming trauma in a lifetime, which changes the meaning of a word for an individual.

For instance, someone who was sacrificed during a celebration in a past life may dread going to a party in this lifetime.

Here are some EFT taps to untangle some of the responses:
(Say each statement three times while tapping on the head with fingertips. Say it a fourth time while tapping on the chest.)

"I release confusing marriage as imprisonment; in all moments."
"I release associating dread with special occasions; in all moments."
"I release associating being beautiful as dangerous; in all moments."
"I release hating children; in all moments."
"I release the trauma of being a parent; in all moments."
"I release associating parenthood with death; in all moments."

"I release confusing success with shame; in all moments."
"I release confusing natural hunger signals as starvation; in all moments."
"I release the fear of starving to death; in all moments."
"I release defining being obese as healthy and safe; in all moments."
"I release associating holidays with sadness and lack; in all moments."
"I release defining nonconformity as dangerous; in all moments."
"I release confusing sugar for love; in all moments."
"I release confusing fatty foods as security; in all moments."
"I release confusing being self-centered as abusing power; in all moments."

These are a few that came through to help uplift the consciousness of the readers this morning.

~ ~ ~ ~ ~

Technique for when you absolutely can't resist that junk food meal:

You know it isn't good for you, you know there is a better choice, but still here you are with this fast food meal in front of you and what are you going to choke it down with? Guilt.

How about realizing that there is something that this meal is providing for you, some kind of love in the form of comfort; use that as a means to bless the meal, and change the vibration of the meal to increase its value.

Put your hands over this meal. Use them like a magnifying glass that concentrates the sun's light rays. Visualize all the love and energy of the cosmos swirling and funneling through your hands and into that meal. Heal whatever was offered up for this meal, bless everyone who worked to bring this meal to you. Thank the rain and the winds and the sunlight for their contribution.

Make the experience so satisfying, so uplifting that it becomes a spiritual moment. Notice how much more easily the meal digests, as if you have just added enzymes and life force to it. You have.

~ ~ ~ ~ ~

One cannot say they have a chronic disease as long as they still ingest:

> processed sugar
> processed meat
> foods with additives and preservatives
> carbonated beverages
> hydrogenated fats and fried foods
> gluten

Until they remove all these ingredients from their diet, they can't consider themselves sick but just responsible for making poor dietary choices.

It takes one from the vantage point of being a random victim to moving to the position of being responsible and empowered.

WEEK 11

We are not martyrs. It is not our moral obligation to suffer an onslaught of tiny assaults under the guise of social obligation. It is not our job descriptions as human beings to suffer insult, lack of appreciation or disrespect at the hands of relatives or friends. We are not meant to diminish ourselves out of an obligatory sense of loyalty.

If going to an event brings more risk than potential gain, it is time to trim the fat on your holiday functions. Dwindle it down to doing only the things that bring mutual joy. Otherwise someone is unnecessarily sacrificing their freedom.

~ ~ ~ ~ ~

Fat Cells Talk Technique:

Have a long heart to heart talk with your fat cells. Thank them for protecting you when you were feeling vulnerable. Tell them that you are strong now and can take care of yourself. Give them permission to shrink down in stature, recede to the background and sleep.

Have a talk with your muscle cells. Give them a pep talk. See them as a little regime of soldiers that have gone soft and undisciplined. Line them up at attention, and see them training to be a strong force in the body. See them as strong marines.

Have a talk with your excretory cells. See them as a waste management company. Have a meeting and tell them that they need to be more efficient. Tell them that they are leaving waste on the streets. Stamp each cell with the little logo of a waste management company so that they know their job.

Have a talk with the public transport system of your body. This is all the veins and arteries carrying blood through the body. Tell them that they have been missing stops on the route and to make sure that every molecule of oxygen is carried to its rightful destination and all toxins are removed from the system.

Have a talk with your heart. Apologize for overworking it and taking it for granted. Explain that you are going to remove the extra fat cells around its encampment and the muscle cells are going to step up to the plate to assist it in doing its job.

~ ~ ~ ~ ~

"I release confusing poverty for humility; in all moments."

It is **NOT OKAY** to make jokes at your own expense. It is **NOT OKAY** to put yourself down and call yourself an idiot, a loser or fat! You are a sacred creation of Love and Light and to put yourself down is to desecrate a beautiful gift. To value yourself is to value all that is good in the world!

WEEK 12

Unharnessing the Slimming Effects of Brown Fat

There are two types of fat. There is the white fat and the brown fat. People who can eat anything they want have more of the brown fat. Many of us would be happy if we had brown fat instead of white fat. The brown fat burns up the white fat for fuel.

Science hasn't found a way to make brown fat more prevalent in the body with a pill, but they have come up with a trick. The trick is to turn the water from hot to cold repeatedly while showering. Since the brown fat is used in mammals to prevent them from freezing during hibernation, the chills hold a key to creating it. So maybe while doing the taps this week, visualize being outside in the winter with almost nothing on. The visual of shivering may create a better conduit to manifest results. Also, since the brown fat is more prevalent in babies, it may be helpful to visualize yourself as an infant as well.

~ ~ ~ ~ ~

My friend said something genius today. She said that the taps that I recently posted about our dynamics with the fat cells was going to just empower the brown fat to seemingly amp her metabolism. Of course, why not? Why not create taps for that?

(Say each statement three times out loud while tapping on you head and say it a fourth time while tapping on your chest.)

"I amp up my metabolism; in all moments."
"I encourage my stem cells to create more brown fat; in all moments."
"I regenerate the production of brown fat in my body; in all moments."
"I make space in my body for more brown fat; in all moments."
"I remove all blockages and limiting beliefs to having more brown fat in my body; in all moments."

~ ~ ~ ~ ~

More Taps for Slimming Effects of Brown Fat

"I stretch my body's capacity to manufacture brown fat; in all moments."
"I recalibrate my body to empower the brown fat; in all moments."
"I awaken and empower my body's brown fat to use up all the white fat; in all moments."
"I command my body to use up all the white fat; in all moments."
"I shift my body's paradigm from white fat to brown fat; in all moments."
"I am centered and empowered in brown fat; in all moments."

When this tap series works for people, they will realize that the other series of taps must work as well. So maybe these particular taps are a key to creating a more health and empowered world. By doing these, we are uplifting humanity one tap at a time.

WEEK 13

Release Being Overweight Marathon

(Say each statement three times out loud while CONTINUOUSLY tapping on the top of your head at the crown chakra, and say it a fourth time while tapping on your chest at the heart chakra. Say each word deliberately. They are not just words but a vibration that you are initiating to shift energy. Pause after each word. Say it in a commanding but even tone, not as a question. Forgo saying it in a sing-song tone or with bravado. Say them all.)

"I release being trapped in a private hell of being overweight; in all moments."
"I release being suffocated by being overweight; in all moments."
"I release identifying with being overweight; in all moments."
"I release calling myself fat; in all moments."
"I release being embedded in the belief that I will always be overweight; in all moments."
"I remove all of being overweight from my beingness; in all moments."
"I release using feelings of being overweight to hide; in all moments."
"I release numbing my feelings to deny being overweight; in all moments."
"I remove all vivaxes between myself and failure to lose weight; in all moments."

"I strip all emotional charge off of being overweight; in all moments."
"I send all energy matrices into the light that support me being overweight; in all moments."
"I heal all the emotional wounds that perpetuate me being overweight; in all moments."
"I remove all the embedded shards of others comments; in regards to being overweight from my beingness; in all moments."
"I release choosing being overweight over my own splendor; in all moments."
"I release denying my own splendor; in all moments."
"I release forgetting my own splendor; in all moments."
"I untangle myself from being overweight; in all moments."
"I remove all vivaxes between myself and being overweight; in all moments."
"I remove all tentacles between myself and being overweight; in all moments."
"I remove the claws of being overweight from my beingness; in all moments."
"I remove all programming and conditioning that being overweight have put on me; in all moments."

~ ~ ~ ~ ~

Marathon Taps Continued

"I remove all engrams that being overweight has put on me; in all moments."
"I remove all limitations that being overweight have put on me; in all moments."

"I remove the illusion of separateness that being overweight have put on me; in all moments."
"I remove the illusion of unworthiness that being overweight have put on me; in all moments."
"I send all energy matrices into the light that contribute to me being overweight; in all moments."
"I send all energy matrices into the light that are devoted to being overweight; in all moments."
"I send all energy matrices into the light that cause me to doubt myself; in all moments."
"I release using being overweight as a crutch; in all moments."
"I release confusing being overweight for security; in all moments."
"I release being paralyzed by being overweight; in all moments."
"I release hiding behind being overweight; in all moments."
"I command all complex matrices to leave and be escorted out by my Guides that contribute to me being overweight; in all moments."
"I remove all symbiotic relationships between myself and being overweight; in all moments."
"I release creating thought forms that contribute to me being overweight; in all moments."
"I extract all thought forms that contribute to me being overweight; in all moments."
"I release spewing negative thoughts about myself into the universal calm; in all moments."
"I release being enslaved to being overweight; in all moments."
"I release enslaving others to regarding me as being overweight; in all moments."

"I release being a binding agent for being overweight; in all moments."
"I release using others as a binding agent for being overweight; in all moments."
"I release being tethered or chained to being overweight; in all moments."
"I release tethering or chaining others to me being overweight; in all moments."
"I free myself of being overweight; in all moments."
"I free all others of seeing me as being overweight; in all moments."
"I recant all vows and agreements between myself and being overweight; in all moments."
"I remove all curses and blessings between myself and being overweight; in all moments."

~ ~ ~ ~ ~

Marathon Taps Continued

"I remove all blessings between myself and being overweight; in all moments."
"I strip all illusion off of being overweight; in all moments."
"I release feeling unable to lose weight; in all moments."
"I release the belief that I am unable to lose weight; in all moments."
"I remove all masks, walls, and armor off of being overweight; in all moments."
"I withdraw all my energy off of being overweight; in all moments."
"I release feeding being overweight; in all moments."

"I sever all strings and cords between myself and being overweight; in all moments."
"I dissolve all karmic ties between myself and being overweight; in all moments."
"I release breathing purpose into being overweight; in all moments."
"I remove all the pain, burden, helplessness, and unworthiness that being overweight has put on me; in all moments."
"I remove all the pain, burden, helplessness, and unworthiness that I have put on all others by being overweight; in all moments."
"I take back all the joy, love, abundance, freedom, health, success and wholeness that being overweight has taken from me; in all moments."
"I give back to all others all the joy, love, abundance, freedom, health, success and wholeness that I have taken from them due to being overweight; in all moments."
"I release resonating with being overweight; in all moments."
"I release emanating with being overweight; in all moments."
"I shift my paradigm from being overweight to being slim and healthy; in all moments."
"I transcend being overweight; in all moments."
"I extract all of being overweight from my sound frequency; in all moments."
"I extract all of being overweight from my light emanation; in all moments."
"I extract all thought-forms of me being overweight from the universal sound frequency; in all moments."

"I extract all thought-forms of me being overweight from the universal light emanation; in all moments."
"I make space in this world to be slim and healthy; in all moments."
"I remove all blockages to me being slim and healthy; in all moments."
"I stretch my capacity to be slim and healthy; in all moments."
"I stretch my capability to maintain being slim and healthy; in all moments."
"I am centered and empowered in being slim and healthy; in all moments."
"I am aligned with the universal image of me being slim and healthy; in all moments."
"I resonate and emanate with being slim and healthy; in all moments."

WEEK 14

EFT Marathon for Food Issues

This is for anyone who has tried every diet and still struggles with food issues. (Say each statement three times while tapping on your head, and say it a fourth time while tapping on your chest.)

I release confusing food for love; in all moments.
I release confusing food for friendship; in all moments.
I release confusing food for fun; in all moments.
I release confusing food for security; in all moments.
I release confusing food for sex; in all moments.
I release confusing food for intimacy; in all moments.
I release confusing food for adventure; in all moments.
I release confusing food for family relationships; in all moments.
I release confusing food for confidence; in all moments.
I release confusing food for a relationship; in all moments.
I release confusing food for power; in all moments.
I release confusing food for success; in all moments.
I release confusing food for companionship; in all moments.
I release confusing food for peace; in all moments.
I release confusing food for likability; in all moments.
I release confusing food for beauty; in all moments.
I release being addicted to food; in all moments..
I release confusing food for friendship; in all moments.

~ ~ ~ ~ ~

EFT Marathon for Food Issues Continued

I shatter the illusion of food; in all moments.
I release using food as a crutch; in all moments.
I release replacing joy with food; in all moments.
I release replacing love with food; in all moments.
I release inhibiting my creativity by eating food; in all moments.
I release trading in my abundance for food; in all moments.
I release choosing food over freedom; in all moments.
I release confusing food for reality; in all moments.
I release choosing food over reality; in all moments.
I release using food as a security blanket; in all moments.
I release allowing food to dumb down my consciousness; in all moments.
I release choosing food over adventure; in all moments.
I release choosing food over life; in all moments.
I release lowering my vibration with food; in all moments.
I release being manipulated by food; in all moments.
I shift my paradigm from food to Joy, Love, Abundance, Freedom, Health, Success, Security, Companionship, Peace, Life, and Wholeness; in all moments.
I release the primal need to forage for food; in all moments.
I release using foraging for food as a distraction from stress; in all moments.
I release mourning my innocence; in all moments.
I release mourning a more innocent time; in all moments.

I release the trauma of starving to death; in all moments.
I release confusing hunger with starving to death; in all moments.
I release the guilt of eating; in all moments.

~ ~ ~ ~ ~

Marathon Taps Continued
I release trying to feed an entire group through my body, in all lifetimes.
I dry up the void of depravity within, in all lifetimes.
I dry up the inner hunger, in all lifetimes.
I release defining being thin as unhealthy, in all lifetimes.
I release associating being thin with disease and poverty, in all lifetimes.
I release the trauma of being poor and diseased, in all lifetimes.
I release associating being this as being invisible, in all lifetimes.
I release confusing being thin with being weak, in all lifetimes.
I release the fear of being weak, in all lifetimes.
I release protecting myself in a big body, in all lifetimes.
I release using weight to compensate for feeling weak, in all lifetimes.
I release confuse carrying extra weight with being strong and safe, in all lifetimes.
I release the fear of being attractive, in all lifetimes.
I release hiding my beauty, in all lifetimes.

I release using weight to hide, in all lifetimes.
I embrace my beauty, in all lifetimes.

WEEK 15

I release eating from boredom; in all moments.
I release eating as a coping mechanism; in all moments.
I release eating because I am sad; in all moments.
I release eating to fill a void; in all moments.
I release eating to feel loved; in all moments.
I release eating to feel comfort; in all moments.
I release eating to feel safe; in all moments.
I release eating to kill time; in all moments.
I release eating to feel busy; in all moments.
I release eating as a form of distraction; in all moments.
I release eating for entertainment; in all moments.
I release eating to be social; in all moments.
I release eating to celebrate; in all moments.
I release thinking of food as a friend; in all moments.
I release the fear of being hungry; in all moments.
I release eating to nurture myself; in all moments.
I release being obsessed with food; in all moments.
I release using food as a hobby; in all moments.
I am centered and satiated in Joy, Love, Abundance, Freedom, Health, Life, and Wholeness; in all moments.

~ ~ ~ ~ ~

I release the fear of being hungry; in all moments.
I release confusing hunger for death; in all moments.
I release going into survival mode when I am hungry; in all moments.
I release defining a huge meal as security; in all moments.
I release defining a huge meal as love; in all moments.

I release confusing sugar for love; in all moments.
I release confusing fatty foods with security; in all moments.
I release the fear of not having enough; in all moments.
I release perceiving mealtime as a competition; in all moments.
I release all the pain and trauma of dying of starvation from my mealtime ritual; in all moments.

~ ~ ~ ~ ~

I release confusing dieting with despair; in all moments.
I release confusing dieting with suicide; in all moments.
I release storing emotional issues in my physical body; in all moments.
I release using my body for emotional storage; in all moments.
I release declaring myself fat; in all moments.
I release eating shame; in all moments.
I release protecting myself in fat; in all moments.
I release insulating myself from pain; in all moments.
I recant all vows and agreements between myself and fat; in all moments.
I remove all curses and blessings between myself and fat; in all moments.
I dissolve all karmic ties between myself and fat; in all moments.
I remove all the pain, burden, and limitations that fat has put on me; in all moments.
I take back all the Joy, Love, Abundance, Freedom, and Wholeness that fat has taken from me; in all moments.

Week 16

Stop Eating Shame

You know when you are eating something that you think that you shouldn't be, you have all those negative thoughts? Well you are kind of eating those feelings and thoughts as a byproduct. Whatever you are eating is being washed down with a side of guilt and shame.

How about coming to terms with whatever you are eating as what you need at that moment for nurturing. Set a conscious intention to turn anything that you are eating, into a positive for eating it. Enjoy the meal. Enjoy the moment.

These Taps will give you the edge for success in being fit:
(Say each statement three times while tapping on your head and say it a fourth time while tapping on your chest.)

"I release eating guilt and shame; in all moments."
"I remove all the guilt and shame that I have ever eaten; in all moments."
"I shift my paradigm from self-loathing to celebrating my own wonder; in all moments."

~ ~ ~ ~ ~

Releasing the Physical Weight of Emotional Pain

There are many reasons why people hold extra weight on their body. In past lives, many of us have starved to death. The relationship with food is so complex. But aside from food issues, people use weight as a means to isolate themselves from the pain of interacting with others.

If someone has been devastated at the hands of others, they may use layers of fat to literally insulate themselves. Since this isn't done on a conscious level, overweight people can obsess over that extra weight. The extra weight can be a direct correlation of the pain they carry from a past life. They are indirectly obsessing over the pain that they are carrying around.

To lose the layers of fat, one may have to let go of the pain that it is storing. The physical weight is reflective of the emotional heaviness. It may be so much more effective to work from the inside first.

"I release storing emotional issues in my physical body; in all moments."
"I release using my body for emotional storage; in all moments."
"I release declaring myself fat; in all moments."
"I release eating shame; in all moments."
"I release protecting myself in fat; in all moments."
"I release insulating myself from pain; in all moments."

~ ~ ~ ~ ~

"I recant all vows and agreements between myself and fat; in all moments."
"I remove all curses and blessings between myself and fat; in all moments."
"I dissolve all karmic ties between myself and fat; in all moments."
I remove all the pain, burden and limitations that fat has put on me; in all moments."
"I take back all the Joy, Love, Abundance, Freedom, and Wholeness that fat has taken from me; in all moments."
"I release resonating with fat; in all moments."
"I release emanating with fat; in all moments."
"I remove all fat from my sound frequency; in all moments."
"I remove all fat from my light body; in all moments."
I shift my paradigm from fat to Joy, Love, Abundance, Freedom, Health and Wholeness; in all moments."

We can use positive affirmation until we are blue in the face. But sometimes, the mind will refute everything positive that we try to manifest for ourselves. It will remind us of how many times we have failed. This is a great technique in sneaking past the mind and making an energetic shift without asking the mind to be on board. The mind does not know how to refute removing fat from the sound frequency. These taps bypass the mind.

WEEK 17

The Riddle Is Solved

Being overweight isn't about being a glutton; it's a clue that your body is out of balance. Cravings are a signal that your body desperately needs something. Since we don't know what the exact thing is, we focus on our default needs like sugar, fat, or just lots of anything.

People who feel a craving for sugar are likely to be in need of love. People who crave fats are most likely in need of security. People who eat a lot are filling a void that may be an actual hole in their energy system. People who are large are trapped in a dualistic schism of being desperate for validation and yet terrified of being seen. None of this is because they are unlovable or even repulsive. But that is what they are resonating with in their energy field, and that is what they manifest to show the world.

Many people, when they eat, feel guilty. They season their food with guilt and eat it. This is one reason diets fail. Instead of learning how to fix the imbalance, we ignore it and starve it. That is what diet is: telling the psyche to shut up and deal with it! This does not fix the underlying issue. This only exacerbates the initial lack.

This process gives tough love to a system that is broken and crying out for kindness. Instead of listening to it, we torture it with deprivation, mute its cries with indifference and even mutilate it to get the results we desire. When the body returns to the image that the broken state reflects, the shame is more intense and the self-defacing behavior is further ingrained.

I never had the heart to go through surgery to mutilate my body by limiting the stomach's holding capacity. I always knew that my hormones and different levels were out of whack. My poor body has been through enough and we are in this together. So I have been doing what I can to heal the primal issues of my body without punishing it, depriving it, or defacing it.

~ ~ ~ ~ ~

Eating to Feel Love

People who eat too much may be using food to pour love into themselves. They are love-starved. Eating food may be the only way they can accept love. This is all very subtle and they may not even understand that this is what they are doing.

When someone tells someone else who is using food to love themselves, that they shouldn't eat so much, they hear that they are not worthy to be loved. That is why it is such a charged issue. The more you try to help them stop eating, the more they are hearing that they are not worth being loved. It happens at a very subtle level.

Cotton Candy Technique

Another technique to satisfy a compulsive desire for food is the cotton candy technique. Since the sun is an important energy supply, visualize the sun as a huge burst of edible energy in the form of cotton candy. During the day, visualize pulling off tufts of sun energy and eating it through the day. Feel it dissolve in your mouth, satiate and energize you. Since action follows thought, you will actually be supplying a deep form of comfort to your body.

~ ~ ~ ~ ~

Coping with Stress and Eating Disorders

Eating is one of the most primal urges. There may be a disconnect between the desire for food in this lifetime and the deprivation of past lifetimes. We forget how vital food is for survival. Even though it seems like a less important need, food for the body is as elemental as the body's need for oxygen.

Compulsive overeaters have experienced starvation in past lifetimes. When they are in binge mode, their brain is in primal mode. The desire to eat overrides mental rational. The same survival mode also overrides the body signals of being full.

A technique to use when someone is a binge eater is to visualize being in the lifetime that they starved in. Imagine feeding THAT body as opposed to the present body. That is why binge eaters never get full; they are not present when they are eating so they never register as full. It's also why the dieting technique of conscious eating is effective. When we're consciously eating, we're bringing our emotional self into the present.

Some of us are so stuck in starvation mode that it's nearly impossible to be present when we eat. We are emotionally trapped in a past experience. The key to overriding this is to consciously bring the food we are presently eating into the other experience. This brings the food we are eating and the hunger we're feeling into alignment. When we aren't consciously eating, it is like bringing food up to your mouth but never having it connect. Bringing the food of the present into the starvation of the past is an empowering technique of feeding the desire behind the food.

Many people vacillate between feeling insecure and sensing the awesome omnipotence of their true self. This creates a skewed self-image. Someone can feel really great about themselves and then look in the mirror and feel Huge. They actually perceive their own energy field. It is much larger than their physical body. If people could separate their energy field from their physical body, they wouldn't feel so confused when they look in the mirror and see a big presence. They would accept the illusion of what they see in the mirror and realize that is good to have a huge presence. It is ridiculous to try to starve an energy field. There is a way to draw in your energy field, but it has nothing to do with food deprivation.

When someone throws up constantly they are really stressed personalities. Food represents energy to them.

Since they have excess energy in the form of stress, they throw up as a way to literally release the stress. There are many techniques to release the stress, but it has nothing to do with food deprivation.

The easiest way to alleviate stress is a collection of techniques that were developed by a man named Lester Levinson. They have developed into two present disciplines. One is called the Sedona Method, and the other is called The Release Technique. Lester Levinson discovered that stress has a weight and a mass. If there were the right intricate machinery, your stress could actually be measured.

Lester taught that stress is trapped energy. It wants to be released. If you want to get rid of stress, just visualize opening up your stomach and your chest and visualize the stress being sucked out by a Universal Vacuum Cleaner. It would look similar to how the air would come rushing out of an opened door on an airplane. Try this technique and see if it helps alleviate stress.

Another technique that is based on the teachings of Lester Levinson is a twist on the vacuum technique. When you are feeling stress being drawn into your lower stomach, it is uncomfortable because it's being stored there until your body can process it. Instead of drawing the stress in, visualize a muscle in the lower stomach blowing the energy out. Developing this sensation and using it can be as simple as changing a setting on your vacuum cleaner.

Once you have figured how to do this, think of things that have caused a stress reaction in your body. At the same time, switch the setting on the stomach to blow the energy out. If you experience a big yawn and a sense of being lighter, you have successfully released your own stress. I believe eating disorders are more about stress and feeling ineffective than about food. The techniques I have suggested are meant to empower.

Check out the Release Technique or the Sedona Method online. Both techniques are proven ways for Healers to stay balanced. I also suggest that you share this message with anyone you know who is stressed or has an eating disorder.

WEEK 18

Chronic Overeating

When someone comes into this lifetime with the unconscious memory of being starved, they may tend to overeat to squelch an insatiable memory. They are trying to reassure their body that it is not going to starve. It is not the physical body that is starving. The memory is so strong that it overrides the physical body cues that it is full.

People who are overweight because of this set themselves up for a cycle of shame by being overweight and starving themselves to compensate. By starving themselves, they are igniting the past life fear and setting themselves up to binge. Also, sugary calories may give the body a similar feeling of emptiness and perpetuate the cycle as well.

That is why a balanced diet is so effective. It may take a long time to reassure yourself, on all levels, that you are not going to starve to death. It is the best way. It takes discipline, but hopefully the awareness that it is a past issue will validate the body in ways junk food cannot.

It may also be good to consciously feed yourself. When you sit down at a meal, get a sense of the lifetime where you were starving and eat from that vantage point. Reassure it that it has come through the lean times and can now be at ease. It's a way of loving yourself. It will hopefully lessen the need to validate that lifetime with hoards of food.

~ ~ ~ ~ ~

An Aversion to Eating

Some people have an aversion to eating. I have uncovered a few of the reasons in my private remote sessions. One of my clients was a food tester for royalty and was poisoned to death. One client's spouse put rat poison in their food and died miserably. One client had to eat rotten food in squalor to survive. Another client starved to death with a whole group of people, so she felt guilty about eating anything at all.

Our body image is so skewed because we are more than a physical body. We have an astral body that is very similar to the physical. Some people can get a sense of it when they look at themselves. You know how there are times when you look in the mirror and you just look so beautiful? This is you seeing the energetic light and love just pouring through yourself. When you look in the mirror and you look distorted or big, you are looking at your astral body and believing it is your physical body. You can do this because you are looking at yourself through your astral eyes.

I know someone who felt so vulnerable in group settings that she made herself really huge as a little girl just so she could be seen. She ended up manifesting a huge physical body for herself. It was not quite the effect that she hoped for since the huge presence made her even more invisible to attention.

The body is fluid, like a river, in the sense that it changes continuously depending on the thoughts and feelings fed to it. If we could realize that we do more good in the world and for ourselves by simply changing our thoughts, we would truly have a grassroots revolution.

~ ~ ~ ~ ~

Here are some taps for people who have an aversion to eating,

I release the fear and trauma of being poisoned; in all moments.
I release the pain and anguish of being poisoned to death; in all moments.
I release the trauma of having to survive in squalor; in all moments.
I release the disgust of eating rotting garbage; in all moments.
I release the guilt of eating when so many have gone hungry; in all moments.
I release trying to starve myself; in all moments.
I release hating food; in all moments.
I release hating myself; in all moments.
I release punishing myself; in all moments.
I release wanting to disappear; in all moments.
I release trying to punish others by starving myself; in all moments.

I release using starving myself to communicate my pain; in all moments.
I release feeling out of control; in all moments.
I release being starved for attention; in all moments.
I release being starved to be heard; in all moments.
I recant my vow of martyrdom; in all moments.
I release being a martyr; in all moments.
I release mourning a past life; in all moments.
I release feeling trapped in an experience; in all moments.
I release using physical and emotional drama to stand out; in all moments.
I release starving to be validated; in all moments.

There are so many varying factors involved in why we do what we do. May these taps give you a clue as to what motivates you on a subliminal level.

WEEK 19

A regular client of mine brought her preschooler to have a session with me. It is so sweet to adapt the work to an age appropriate level. The girl would not eat. She was very fussy and random about what she would and would not eat.

In the past, there were no forensics, so a very convenient way to eliminate someone was by poisoning them. So I led the little girl through the EFT tap, "I release being poisoned." It seemed to help. The eating issue resolved itself.

It made me wonder if some eating disorders are a result of a similar issue in the past. I know part of the compulsion for people to will themselves to throw up is that they are so congested with stagnant energy that they are trying to remove the pain by convulsing it out. Some clients have had the experience of seeing themselves throwing up a stream of black sludge. Maybe some bulimics are stuck in the trauma of being poisoned in a past life.

Some of the issues that people are having may be better addressed by looking at their past and tuning into a deeper cause rather than labeling the issues under one heading such as "food issues."

~ ~ ~ ~ ~

Binge Eating

A woman had trouble with binge eating. It was a terrible problem. When she ate, she would go on automatic pilot, and she never got full. It was so bad that she would get physically sick before she would register as full.

In a past life, she lived in a village where there was no food. When she ate, she felt guilty because it transported her to a time when everyone around her was starving. Not only was she trying to feed the emaciated body she once had, she was trying to eat for the whole village. The shame she was feeling wasn't as much about eating too much, it was about shame that she was eating at all when others were starving.

Understanding her past was the beginning of separating the past from the present. This is a reason why the practice of conscious eating is so important. It keeps one grounded in the present, so the present body registers getting fed.

A great technique to use if one is a binge eater:

Imagine a scenario where the people are all hungry. Anything that you imagine will be a familiar scenario for you. Visualize going into the scenario with truckloads of food. Imagine feeding every last one of the people in the scenario. Go through the process of feeling every last member satiated and full.

Try doing this technique before every meal. Change up the scenarios if you get tired of one or another one presents itself. Mock up different time periods that starvation occurred.

Also try these EFT taps:

I release the devastation of starving to death; in all moments.
I release confusing hunger with imminent death; in all moments.
I satiate every aspect of my beingness; in all moments.

~ ~ ~ ~ ~

Unlocking the Code

Some people are struggling right now with their issues, mindsets and lives. Anything that anyone is thinking, feeling or experiencing is temporary. They can just pass right through it if they will do the opposite of what they are compelled to do.

When people are stuck in their mind grooves, they think and feel a certain way and believe it is reality. It is no different than someone being in a deep ditch and thinking that life is all about living in the ditch. They try to pull others into the ditch because they are lonely, desperate and want to be validated. This is indulgent.

I have become very intolerant of people pulling others into the ditch. Many good people are doing what they can to stay balanced and because of their compassion they may open up to someone who seems to need help.

But no one can help another unless they are first centered and balanced themselves and equipped to handle these experts at pulling.

The reality is that no one can help another unless that person is ready to climb out of the ditch. It is a waste of energy to try. If people still watch the news and are obsessed with what is wrong in the world, they are responsible for what they allow in. This world is a tough training ground for the strengthening of the human spirit, but anyone who reads this has enough tools at their fingertips to assist themselves in having a balanced life.

WEEK 20

Here is a checklist of things to do to stay centered:

Turn off the news and current events. It is a stream of negative consciousness meant intentionally to draw people into drama.
Connect with a higher source every day, every moment possible.
Wean yourself off processed foods as much as your budget will allow, especially sugar. Bless the food that you eat as love and gratitude are powerful enzymes.
Take vitamins and minerals to enrich the physical body.
Perform some kind of physical activity everyday.
Perform some kind of creative venture to engage the mind.
Listen only to uplifting music.
Get rid of negative thoughts by writing them out or putting them in a bubble of light and sending them away. (Please think responsibly by not dumping them on others.)
Perform a kindness each day for someone other than yourself. You are your worst enemy when you are focused totally on yourself.
Say thank you often, especially for the ability to breath, eat, laugh, walk, dance, play, speak your mind, engage others freely. These are all gifts that some don't have, and many who do, take for granted.
Stay focused in the moment at hand. There is only the moment. The rest is only an illusion.

These things are the bare basics of survival. Make a chart of the days of the week with a checklist box next to every one. Stick it on the refrigerator and check off the items every day as you do them. (Don't forget to be grateful that you have a refrigerator.) Add your own items to the list.

~ ~ ~ ~ ~

This life is about figuring out how to give your gifts. It may seem difficult, but sometimes the people with the most reason to complain and resent their life are the ones that serve others. Why is that? They have cracked the code. Life is about others. Life is about loving and serving and gratitude and joy. "Be the love that you want to see in the world" isn't a trite statement. It is the combination to unlocking all the Joy, Love, Abundance and Freedom that the world has to offer. Godspeed.

~ ~ ~ ~ ~

Triggers

When figuring out what people are allergic to, the doctor will remove all potential causes from their diet and add one item at a time to their diet to see what the reaction is. This is a great technique to use in keeping your life balanced as well.

When starting this endeavor, it will be difficult to catch all the contaminants for yourself. But the key is getting to a point of emotional and mental balance so that you can take note of every thing happening in your environment that brings dis-ease. A good time to start is the first thing in the morning.

When you wake up, pay attention to your mood. If it is a good one, start removing the triggers as they come. If it isn't a good one, you may want to look at the triggers from the night before. Sometimes foods and interactions the night before can cause a reaction, so these are things you can look at with that awareness.

For example, if you have eaten a certain food the night before or watched a scary movie, and had a nightmare, you may know enough to avoid those so as not to have the same effect. Use this technique to comb through everything that is causing the slightest discomfort. You will get to the point where you can control every situation and environmental cause that seemed impossible a short time before. Or at least know what is bringing them out of balance.

When you wake up in a peaceful state, it is an easy place to stay mindful of not feeling peaceful. The first sign that your mood is changing, make a note of what is transpiring at that moment. That is a means of figuring out the once unconscious triggers. And some of them are subtle. It can be something as innocuous as wearing polyester. (Believe it or not, this is a big one). Or an outfit you wore when you were in a bad mood and didn't wash yet. That is how subtle triggers can be.

Other triggers are certain people, music, watching television or certain shows, certain scents, activities that trigger unpleasant events, problems not dealt with, etc. Triggers are basically anything you think, feel, say, do, anyone you interact with or don't interact with, anything that engages any of the five senses or even the lack of stimulant. The more you are mindful of and able to eliminate the unconscious triggers, the more conscious you can live. It will also help you get a better handle on the triggers that you thought you could not control, like other people, their circumstances and even dis-ease.

WEEK 21

The Physiology Exchange of Emotional Energy

It's common sense that if we drink a lot of water, we will have to relieve our bladder at some point of that water. But when it comes to ingesting anger, sadness, and other "heavy" emotions, we think that they are just magically transformed. Because we can't see them, we disconnect from the process of relieving them. Yet our verbiage tells us otherwise.

"Someone dumped on me today."
"I just had to talk it out."
"I have to bounce it off someone."
"I am taking in everything that you are saying."

We know that there is a need to get rid of these issues. The lazy way is to dump them onto some agreeable soul. This is pure ignorance to continue to do so. People are hurting their friends because they are too lazy to take action to convert the stagnant energy into a more productive form. Of course, some people are in a chronic state and may need help of a professional who is equipped to deal with their barrage of emotional energy. But the rest of us should not be made to feel guilty by not being dumping grounds for a friend's issues. That should not be the requirement of a friend or a commonality in friendship.

~ ~ ~ ~ ~

There are so many people who say they love their friends but have to limit their time with them because all the friend does is talk about their problems. The friend will even get angry with the person who tries to pull back and ask why the person cut them off. The person is cutting the friend off out of self-preservation. It is a necessary survival tool sometimes.

There are more self-responsible ways to convert this energy from stagnant emotional energy to something productive.

Journal - It is a safe and effective way of getting emotions out.
Exercise - It converts emotional energy into kinetic energy.
Self Improvement - It is converting negative energy into positive energy.
Helping others - The feel-good component will override the resistance that the stored issues will invoke.
(That is all resistance is: stagnant emotional issues that want to stay put.)

Just realizing that there is an exchange of energy in every interaction will make people more conscious and responsible as to what they bring to the table. For example, the reason people get irritable when they are dieting is because all the anger that they stored in the liver is now being separated from the fat they stored and is now manifesting in the state in which it came to the individual. How many overweight people have situations in their life that are overwhelming? Being overweight isn't about being greedy for food; it is about needing a base substance of fat to store the emotional issues that are being carried. People are eating their problems.

People need to be trained how to treat each other. When some people secure a session with me, they think they will be dumping all their angst onto me. I cannot allow that. When I try to explain that I cannot process all the emotions that they want to pass over, that I merely unhook them from their problems and send the problems away, they feel frustrated and may continue to energetically vomit on me. I consider it rude at some point, and if they continue, may choose not to interact with them in the future. It is not honoring an agreement to dump on others. My way is effective. Their way may serve them, but it doesn't serve their target victim, the friend.

~ ~ ~ ~ ~

Some people look for horrific things to put on their status page. They know they are affecting others. It makes them feel important. People know that it feels good to unload on their page because good people are reading it and taking it in for them. They are disconnected by the cause and affect of their actions and just went with the feel-good component of it.

If you are someone who people find to dump on, you may want to look at that. It may feel good short-term to listen to someone and make them feel good. But how does it serve you in the long run? Is your life running smoothly? How is your health? I guarantee that many of the people who have fibromyalgia are the caring, nurturing types. I have told a few of them to purge from nurturing others for a while. But they have been incapable of doing that because that is how their sense of self is being fed.

If you are being dumped on share this. The next time someone starts to dump, stop them and shift to something neutral. Explain that it doesn't feel good to your well-being to listen to their problems. If they understand, then they care about you. If they react, they are inadvertently using you for their own well-being. If they continue, tell them to please stop and continue to advocate for yourself by telling them to shut up if you have to. Make the distinction between caring about them but not caring about hearing their issues. If they still continue, you may have to cut them off. Your well-being and your sense of wholeness is your first priority. It is your first job in life to maintain your own balance. Your happiness and sense of balance is never on the table as a bargaining chip for friendship. But a friend's respect of your boundaries and a sense of responsibility in interacting with you are on the table. You hold all the cards. Play your hand wisely!

WEEK 22

Utilizing the Dream State for Self-Growth

Many people think that dreams are random. This is not my truth. Dreams are our higher wisdom's attempts to awaken us. But there is a curtain between this life and our wholeness that prevents us from being overwhelmed here by the vastness of our experiences. The curtain that divides the states of awakening and our physical existence divide as much as they need to. The more we are committed to delving into ourselves, the more we will be shown. For some, it is a thin veil that divides the two states.

I never share my dreams. But I was guided to do that with a dream that I woke up from to show others how to carry the information of the dreams into their contemplative state to empower themselves.

In my dream, the town was in a frenzy. It was terrified about running out of food. As I was walking over the bridge into town, I noticed there were feces next to the river. The porta potties were filled so people were defecating next to them. The river was contaminated as well.

In town, the supermarket was in a frenzy. The shelves were being emptied, and everyone was in chaos. I walked around calmly. The deli clerk offered me some item, and I politely refused. I was calm and non-reactive.

When I awoke, I immediately knew what this dream was about for me. It was a message for me. Not some generic person but for me. It was utilizing all my experiences to show me an aspect of me a little better.

Here is what my dream means to me: Since I was starved nearly to death a few years ago, it has been difficult for me to suppress the urge to eat. If I get hungry, it creates a panic attack in me. The same has been true with exercise. Doing either creates the trauma that existed in me during that year of captivity. The frenzied people in the dream are my cells. They are panicking because I have been successfully dieting for the last five months. They are terrified of being starved to death. Also, the feces means all the toxins that my body is dumping more quickly than the river can carry them away. But my higher awareness walked around the store knowing that everything will be fine. It was calm and nonreactive.

Using this information, I can improve my state of affairs in contemplation. In a quiet time, I merely go to the town and reassure all the town's people (which are the cells of my body) that they will not go hungry. I replace all the bakery items on the shelf with vitamins and water that are very filling and plentiful. I visualize everyone calming down and being happy with the lighter improvements to the local diet. I see everyone working and productive and happy. I see the feces (which represents byproducts and toxins of losing weight) being cleaned up and the river washing away and clear. I visualize the sun shining, everyone happy and productive, many children playing and laughing and everyone satisfied.

~ ~ ~ ~ ~

Any dream that you have reveals the ability to recreate yourself in your desired state. This is not random. It is a tool for all to use. Some will say that they don't remember their dreams, but it is because the indifference made them stop looking at them. Tell yourself before you go to sleep at night to remember your dreams. And when you wake up, figure out how to use the information that you have been given to improve your quality of life.

~ ~ ~ ~ ~

Even the person who says that they don't dream at all will invite their dreams to manifest with the intention to write them down. To keep a pen and paper handy to jot down any memories that are bleeding through is a huge conduit for bridging the awareness between the awakened and sleeping state. If you practice writing down your dreams regularly, you may soon wonder which is really the dream state and which is the awakened state.

WEEK 23

Perpetual contemplation

Everything we do can be done in a meditative or contemplative state to bring more love and awareness into our lives. The key is simply doing it with more conscious intention.
For example:

When you are bathing, you can visualize washing away negative thought forms from yourself.

When you speak, you can think of each word as a burst of positive or negative energy that you are adding into the environment. You can speak with the intention of only adding positive energy to the whole.

When you are driving home, you can feel the communion of all the other drivers and treat them with the reverence of leaving church.

~ ~ ~ ~ ~

Perpetual contemplation

When you eat, you can visualize the love being extracted out of the food and sending it to all the cells of your body. You can send gratitude back to the sponsors of your meal: the earth and the plants.

When anything unusual happens during the day, you can treat it like a dream message and interpret its meaning.

When you are doing something that you don't enjoy, visualize how much worse conditions may have been in past eras and be grateful for the contrast.

When you are relaxing, imagine yourself resting in the arms of love.

~ ~ ~ ~ ~

Perpetual contemplation

When someone offers you anything uplifting, see it as a gift from the Universe and accept graciously.

When you are walking your dog, you can realize how they feel when they are enjoying their favorite pastime and allow the pet the space to enjoy themselves unhindered by control.

When you love your children, you can imagine yourself as a child as well and realize it is nurturing yourself by nurturing them.

This is a way to make the whole day richer and to enliven the lives of those around us more than we already do.

WEEK 24

The Answer on Drug Use...Intention

Recently, I facilitated a private remote session with a regular client. She is struggling with the moral and physiological issue of smoking marijuana. I had to cancel a previous session with her because she was high at the time. She was really confused as to why it was an issue. I tried to explain to her why I did not want to facilitate a sessions with her if she was committed to smoking marijuana.

When I am doing energy work, I am receptive and open. I have to be so acute in my awareness and at the same time protect myself from foreign energies. When someone indulges in smoking, drinking, rich foods, or drugs, it is many times, foreign energies that are compelling one to indulge. It is like being home and having all the doors and windows of your house open where anyone can walk in. Before I do work with anyone, they need to have the intention of closing all their windows and doors. Otherwise, the point of me helping is moot. It would be like trying to convert a gang of thugs.

She had a sincere question as to why marijuana was not good for her. I had no answer for her really except that it pokes holes in your energy field, and I don't feel comfortable working with anyone who is actively participating. But to her, smoking marijuana was spiritual. In her session, I received the answer she needed.

In her past lives, I saw her using herbs in spiritual ritual. I saw her smoking the peace pipe, and I saw her drinking an ambrosia in an ancient Aztec-like culture. These drugs took her to a spiritually higher consciousness. It was a good memory that she relived by smoking marijuana in the present.

But then I saw the marijuana of the present and how it is used to subjugate the masses. I saw the drug trades, sex trafficking, the buying and selling of guns to dangerous militia groups all funded and run by the money made in drug sales. I saw people being literally led down a beautiful wooded path that felt spiritual and wonderful, but as it went on longer and grew wider, it became a tarred-over smelly mining road. It just kept going and going and the people who were on it were too tired to go back but realized that they were walking to a wasteland. That is where drug use literally takes people.

So I received the answer to my client's question, "Why were drugs okay in past life experiences but not okay in the present climate?" The answer is intention. In the past, the smoking of a drug took the client to a higher vibration where she could connect with her spiritual self. In the present, smoking marijuana led her to a lie because she was not led anywhere good in the smoking of it. She was merely pacified while she denied expressing her own greatness. It was not medicinal for her. It was a crutch.

Where recreational drugs lead now is a cesspool. The consciousness of a person these days is that they can get beyond their own limitations much easier without indulging in the lie that drugs are helping them. People will argue this with me but they are being duped. I see the illusion of where drugs empty the person out in the other worlds. It is very low in the worlds of God. Very low. I would never stop there even to get a drink except if I was helping someone who was trapped there, which I was.

~ ~ ~ ~ ~

The woman just mentioned felt that she had demons. That was her excuse to give away her power. She had no demons. The energy she felt was stagnant energy within her creating a personification of itself and lying to her. It was dead energy that she gave life to with her fear and her beliefs. It was time for her to do some inner dusting and take back her power.

(Say each statement three times out loud while continuously tapping on the top of your head at the crown chakra and say it a fourth time while tapping on your heart Chakra

"I release harboring demons; in all moments."
"I release sympathizing with my demons; in all moments."
"I release feeding my demons; in all moments."
"I release giving power over to my demons; in all moments."
"I release creating demons; in all moments."

"I release the fear of my own demons; in all moments."
"I release giving my demons super human strength; in all moments."
"I release the belief that my demons are evil spirits; in all moments."
"I release confusing my demons with demonic possession; in all moments"
"I exorcise my demons; in all moments."
"I release owning the demons; in all moments."
"I release being enslaved to the demons; in all moments."
"I recant all vows and agreements between myself and the demons; in all moments."
"I remove all blessings and curses between myself and the demons in all moments."
"I sever all strings and cords between myself and the demons; in all moment."
"I am centered and empowered in divine love; in all moments."
"I remove and dissolve everything from my beingness that is not divine love; in all moments."
"I resonate and emanate divine love; in all moments."

~ ~ ~ ~ ~

"I break all chains between myself and the demons; in all moments."
"I dissolve all karmic ties between myself and the demons; in all moments."
'I remove all the fear, guilt, pain, burden, limitations, anger, greed, lust, jealousy and engrams that the demons have put on me; in all moments."

"I take back all the joy, love, abundance, freedom, health, success, security, companionship, peace, life, wholeness, beauty, enthusiasm, contentment, spirituality, enlightenment and confidence that the demons have taken from me; in all moments."
"I withdraw all my energy from the demons; in all moments."
"I collapse and disintegrate the demons into divine love; in all moments."
"I repair and fortify the Wei Chi of all my bodies; in all moments."
"I align all my bodies; in all moments."
"I release resonating with the demons; in all moments."
"I release emanating with the demons; in all moments."
"I extract all the demons from my sound frequency and dissolve them into divine love; in all moments."
"I extract all the demons from my light body and dissolve them into divine love; in all moments."
"I shift my paradigm from the demons to joy, love, abundance, freedom, health, success, security, companionship, peace, life, wholeness, beauty, enthusiasm, contentment, spirituality, enlightenment and confidence; in all moments."
"I transcend the demons; in all moments."
"I am centered and empowered in divine love; in all moments."
"I remove and dissolve everything from my beingness that is not divine love; in all moments."
"I resonate and emanate divine love; in all moments."

WEEK 25

Fat Shaming

The truth of the matter is that your outer appearance is so insignificant compared to your inner work. Putting so much emphasis on the outer appearance is another form of societal control. It is another way to make someone feel diminished and unfulfilled. There are infinite reasons that people overeat. One is that they have starved to death in past lives. The fear of starvation is registered in their DNA. If it takes a lifetime of overeating to reassure themselves that the experience is over, then that is what they need to do.

Someone who is overweight is using it at a coping mechanism. To shame them is to take someone who is coping with pain and shove more pain into them. Why is that not considered cruel? It is like telling a person who is doing the best that they can and is coping in the only way they know that they are unworthy and undesirable because of it. It is a form of abandonment. It can be just as silly and unwarranted as shaming someone who has come back from war for having post-traumatic stress disorder.

~~~~~

Here are just some of the reasons for being overweight or overeating:

Starving in a past life.
Modern foods are engineered to make you fatter as an illusion to make humans seem fulfilled.
Modern foods are engineered to make you hungrier to sell more products.
Advertisements brainwash people to eat more.
Social situations center around indulgence.
Binging can be reverting to a peaceful primal lifetime of being a gatherer.
Trying to feed an aspect of yourself that starved in a past lifetime.
Guilt over being able to eat when others have starved, and you are trying to feed a whole village indirectly.
Keeping layers of fat on you as a form of protection.
Wanting to be undesirable so you don't get sacrificed for your beauty.
Wanting to be undesirable because you have been raped and abused in past times.
A form of hiding in plain sight.
Associating sugar with love.
Associating fat with security.
Associating eating itself with a bonding of your people.
(In past times people ate big feasts when they were not at war and it was safe to do so.)
Grounding your energy so that you feel like you aren't floating away.
Feeling heavy as a way to feel like you do indeed exist and are not invisible.
A way to empower yourself by making your energy big so no one can hurt you.
Fear of not existing.

Memories of eating with a group and trying to reconnect to that experience.
A way to store issues into yourself because you don't want to hurt someone else.
People realizing that it may be their last lifetime to eat food so they are taking in as much of the experience as possible.

These are some of the reasons. There is nothing here about being disgusting or greedy or not caring about oneself. The issue of eating and weight is a very painful experience for the individual. Shaming them is jamming more pain into them. Shaming them is a form of ignorance.

~ ~ ~ ~ ~

In past times, people worked so hard that they needed foods to be hearty. In modern times food has taken on the roll of entertainment. To some of us, it would be easier if we could quit eating altogether like other vices. But food is a primal need like water and air.

Perhaps we can evolve as a species to be able to ingest energy directly from source and not need to eat food at all. Until that happens, just please be kind to others. Just because you can see they are struggling with something, doesn't mean that it is more than someone else is dealing with. It just means that their struggle is more obvious. To kick someone when they are struggling is ignorance at its best.

WEEK 26

Transcending Eating Meat

With the greatest minds and all the savvy technology that we have, a few bright researchers must have stumbled upon the correlation between dis-ease and physical health: There is a direct relationship between the emotional component and a physical disease. Maybe they have realized that emotional issues have literal mass and can break down the integrity of the DNA strand, so even genetic diseases are affected by emotional components.

But some savvy minds with an agenda must have reached further into the understanding to realize that we treat our meat sources like crap. We pull them away from their mother, show them no physical kindness, pen them in crates that are too small to even turn around in or lay down, even when they are pregnant and expect that terror not to affect the human when they ingest it.

We imply very generally that eating meat is unhealthy. When it is more an understanding amongst people who study these things that the trauma, brutality and insanity that we inflict on the sweet animals that provide us protein is stored in their tissue as memory. When we ingest the animal meat, we are not just eating a lifeless protein. We are taking in a life force. Native Americans understand this and that is why they honor the kill that they have taken down.

But every day, millions of Americans are ingesting the life force of a deranged and broken beast whose feelings and well being were twisted into such a state of horror that nothing humane is left in them when they are walked into the rendering plant. The memory of that horror lives on in the humans that eat it. That is the curse that we have inflicted on ourselves by treating our brethren of the earth so unjustly.

I have heard people rationalize that it is animals' soul contract to be used as food. Perhaps. But whatever we inflict on them as caretakers is our soul contract to then bear. Have we agreed to subject ourselves to such trauma?

I have had the experience of walking into that rendering plant as the cow and experienced the sights and sounds of being methodically butchered. I have felt the anguish in my hamburger of the systemic indifference of how beautiful, kind and loving creatures are murdered. I have struggled with this awareness as I choke down the meat that my body has craved and that has become a ritual of every holiday in the book; that I am ingesting pure suffering. I crave the barbecue from afar. But when it is placed before me, my body rejects the reality of it.

A natural byproduct of my sensitivities has become the inability to ingest meat. It literally chokes me the times that I still try. I have done mass healings on the herds and flocks that it came from; I have altered the vibration with intention, but still my body reacts to the suffering that the meat has endured. No human wants to suffer, yet they so readily eat second hand suffering daily. They do not realize what they are storing up in their own atoms. It is something that the body wholeheartedly rejects.

The vibrations of the world are changing. The rules are changing as well. If you are someone that accepted meat easily into your body and enjoyed it, but are having indigestion problems, health issues or emotional imbalances for no apparent reason, you may want to address your diet. We are becoming too sensitive as human beings to repeatedly ingest so much misery into our systems on a daily basis. You can stay in denial all you want, and still the misery and horror that the animals you ingest will be a part of your reality. It is a simple transference. You are what you eat.

~ ~ ~ ~ ~

The lobbyists for meat spend billions on funny commercials about bacon, bacon and more bacon. They care as little about your health as they do the welfare of the animals that are owned by filthy rich billionaires who can buy an agenda as easily as you buy gum. They are manipulating and twisting reality to fit their needs. Their need is for everyone to keep consuming animal meat even though it is a lose-lose for animal and human. If you get sick, no problem to them, they most likely have stock in some medical establishment that will get your money as the human bodies break down from the onslaught of emotional trauma.

You are your only advocate. If you are aware, you can pay attention to exactly how you feel after you eat meat and know for your self that feeling of not being comfortable in your skin is caused by the meat you eat. You will be able to pull away from the social pressure to eat meat and do what is best for you. It is when more and more people opt out from being conditioned to indifference that an effective change will be made.

In the past, people have been unable to correlate how they feel with the quality of their food. It is no longer a moral issue but a self-serving one. That is how corrosive the meat you eat has become. Now perhaps, with the awareness that it is indeed affecting people's health and well being, a change can now be made.

A diet of the future will entail only things that are giving graciously. Fruits, nuts and legumes are all gracious givers. Perhaps at one time, the families' livestock would willingly give themselves over for the love that the families were giving. But that exchange has become antiquated, and perhaps with it, the ability to easily digest meat.

~ ~ ~ ~ ~

"I heal all those I have ingested; in all moments."
"I make whole all that I have eaten; in all moments."
"I honor the spirit of all those who have sustained me;

in all moments.
"I release the trauma of all those I have ingested in indifference; in all moments."
"I release carrying the weight of all those I have ingested; in all moments."
"I free myself from the plague of indifference in regards to all food supplies; in all moments."
"I exonerate myself in regards to all food supplies; in all moments."

WEEK 27

Engrams

Have you ever been going through your day and a memory just pops through of doing something in the past? That is an engram. An engram is a tiny ridge in your energy field similar to ridges in an old vinyl record. The record will play a song when the groove is stimulated by the needle of the stereo. In a similar way, our engrams will be stimulated by a thought or experience, sight or smell that is similar to the one in the engram.

For example, if you have gotten sick by eating a certain food, you may be reminded of that feeling every time you are presented with that food. It will give you an aversion to eating that food again. This is very beneficial in figuring out the ways we have come to our physical demise in a past life.

People who are afraid of, or have an aversion to a certain something, most likely died in that way or some way similar. For example, someone who is afraid of heights most likely has fallen to their death in a past life. So when they get near a place where they could fall, that memory is triggered and they are afraid. This is good to know because most fears are a memory of things that have already happened. So there is really little fear of looming disaster. If people can wrap their mind around this, they can relinquish many of their fears. It is very empowering.

These engrams are triggered all the time within us. When we have a reaction that comes out of the blue, most likely an engram is being triggered. There are also pleasant engrams, too. People, places and things can all trigger engrams--even and especially family members. Your relationship with your family was most likely forged in past times. So there is no need to feel flawed if you don't fit in. Most likely, you were an outsider to them in a past time. Perhaps even a slave or a prisoner that they incurred through war.

~ ~ ~ ~ ~

There are universal engrams that one can recognize in others.

When someone has an aversion to religion they most likely suffered at the hands of austere practices within a sect.

Those who have an aversion to the Roman Catholic Church, many times fought and died in the crusades.

Those who come back gay, many times have suffered in the body of the opposite sex that they were in. Their torment was so severe that they have an aversion to coming back as that sex again. But there are still lessons to learn as that sex. So the body comes back as if they were in that opposite sex and are attracted to the persons they would in that body. To understand this is to also understand why it is incredibly heartless to judge gay people for their experiences. The assault they have already endured may have been tremendous.

Many times, people who come back eager to serve as soldiers have been many times. It is a form of a habit to serve. Perhaps the poor treatment many soldiers have experienced from society and the government in this life is enough to smooth down that engram, so in future lives they are no longer compelled to serve out of duty.

Those who feel unworthy are perhaps triggering a lifetime when they were an untouchable, when countries still had the caste system.

Many people who are hopelessly uninspired and non-productive may be healing from a past lifetime at war, and they are doing the best that they can.

There are many many reasons to be compassionate to yourself and others.

~ ~ ~ ~ ~

The key to empowerment is to be aware of these engrams when they occur so you are not living in reactionary mode. It is possible to "rub out" these engrams so that you are only left with the pleasant ones: Be kind and loving to yourself and others in every situation and stay aware. These are ways to rub out engrams.

I assisted a family that was having trouble with their children. They were a well-structured family with great kids, but consistently after dinner, the children would break down and become very moody. Both parents had stressful jobs so I knew intuitively what was happening.

The parents would come right home and start making dinner. Making dinner was used as a way to transition from workday to family. Then the family would sit down and talk about their days.

The mother was unconsciously putting all her angst from the day into the food she was preparing for her family. She felt great, but the children were eating what she unloaded. Also, at the table, the children had to listen to all these adult problems and interactions that their parents were dealing with. The parents felt great after this family ritual, but the children were absorbing all the angst that they had just downloaded.

What I suggested for the parents is that when they get home from work to slip into a quiet room for a half hour before interacting with the children. They should do a slight meditation, visualization or even listen to music and let the chords of music carry away the stress. Then, and only then, should they interact with their children.

I also suggested that when they cooked, they were conscious to put good intentions into the food and make that be the focus of meal. And limit all conversation at the table to what went right about the day, what lessons were learned, who did they help, what did they witness that was uplifting.

This change in their day saved their children from wilting under the weight of having parents with stressful positions.

WEEK 28

Being Beautiful

I recently facilitated a session with an attractive woman who believed she wasn't beautiful. This is such a common belief. For some, being beautiful translates to happiness.

This issue ran very deep. The surface belief is that she wasn't attracting happiness in the form of a loving relationship because she wasn't beautiful enough. Her past lives showed me how she was so mistreated in past lives that she correlated relationships with abuse. Physical features were not a factor.

She lived in times when most women were abused and treated poorly, called horrible names and degraded. In a past life, she saw a beautiful woman that seemed respected and sought after. From that vantage point that woman seemed to have happiness, and that is how she correlated beauty with happiness. It meant not being abused and unappreciated.

I have facilitated other sessions where women who were beautiful had such an aversion to it because they were sacrificed to the Gods for being the most beautiful. One woman correlated beauty and adulation with fear and distrust. She happily creates a "plain Jane" persona. To her, that is peace and contentment.

In the session with the first woman, her mother, who had crossed, came through and stroked her face and gave her a pep talk. Her little grandmother came through as well to remind her how special she is. Sometimes, loved ones on the other side seem to help their living loved one (even loving pets) make a connection with me as a means to either give them a message or to just help them. This seemed to be one of those instances.

So many people waste so much energy in thinking and believing badly about themselves. If they could only accept that who they are and how they react is all formulated by their experiences and their unconscious fears and aversions. Then people would accept that they are doing the best they can to take care of their own needs and stop making themselves suffer more as a survival tactic.

~ ~ ~ ~ ~

Here are some taps I created to help:
(Say each statement three times while tapping on the head and say it a fourth time while tapping on the chest)

"I release the aversion to being beautiful; in all moments."
"I release correlating beauty with happiness; in all moments."
"I release the trauma of being sacrificed; in all moments."
"I release being invisible; in all moments."
"I release feeling unworthy; in all moments."

"I release the belief that I am undesirable; in all moments."
"I release burying my gifts; in all moments."

May these releases help women who choose to mute their own beauty through a lack of self-care or by putting on layers of weight as a means to hide.

~ ~ ~ ~ ~

Cleaning the Body's Filter

The liver filters out fat and toxins from the body. It also filters the subtle energies that are released when one facilitates energy work. It is important to cleanse the filter just as it is important to clean the filter of the dryer. If one has trouble losing weight, feels tired after interactions with others, or has a pain in the upper right side of their torso, they may want to cleanse the liver.

A great way to clean the liver is by eating pomegranates. Pomegranates are naturally astringent and cut through the mucus. They burn more calories than they contain in eating them. Also, they have a property that actually regenerates liver tissue. Since they are food, there are no side affects to using this as a cleanse.

To eat them, gently peel the outside without breaking the little pearls of flesh inside. There will be sections of pearls inside. Gently pull apart the sections and gently eat the pearls of flesh. They may stain your fingers or clothes, but it is well worth it to benefit from their healing properties.

WEEK 29

Seven Billion Balloons

There is a technique that says, answer these three questions before you say anything: Is it true? Is it necessary? Is it kind? If a statement passes all three criteria then it is worthy of speaking.

I use this gauge to monitor thoughts as well. I dissolve the thoughts that don't meet this criteria. This applies to thoughts about ourselves as well. This is a good baseline assessment of what is worth manifesting in thoughts as well as in speech.

After this test is mastered, I use the weight test. I weigh my words in my mind. Negative words are heavy such as war, disease and negative descriptive words. Uplifting words are light. That is why that are called uplifting. They literally uplift consciousness through their utterance. I think and say only words that are uplifting.

You are beautiful, you are wonderful, you are amazing are all uplifting statements. They are true as well. When we say positive statements that we mean, there is such a dynamic energy to them. When we speak truth, it is the difference between holding a beautiful crystal with healing properties instead of a piece of glass.

It is a real art form to convey world issues accurately in uplifting words. For some, it may be difficult to stop unconsciously talking, and for some it may be difficult to stop going on about problems and the plight of the world. It may be very difficult to convey our personal issues in uplifting words. But it can be done. Wouldn't that be a great way to know what is worthy to be shared? If it can be conveyed in uplifting terms, than it is okay to manifest. What a great exercise and personal challenge.

Maybe each person's words are like a balloon that is able to uplift humanity or weigh it down, but not enough for the individual to move the whole thing. Maybe all of us collectively have been weighing humanity down with the disregard for our responsibility in this matter. But maybe if each one of us elevates our thoughts and our speech, each one could be like a helium balloon. When the multitudes of individuals each learn to elevate their personal thoughts and speech, they will be like a huge bunch of helium balloons. In this way, we can all do our part to uplift humanity.

~ ~ ~ ~ ~

Taps of the Day

Eliminating the Initial Cause of Pain

In the game of Dominoes, that first tile is so important. If the first domino was not there, the whole chain reaction would not occur. It is this way in life as well. Have you ever done something that set off a whole chain of reactions. It was so devastating that the results were life changing and not in a good way? You so wish you could take that one course of events back?

This is how it goes in the way of life as well. At one point, we were so full of joy, love, beauty, health, and abundance. We were also all free and whole. But then that one instance happened in our repertoire of experiences that caused us to veer a little bit from the absolute best. It was the first thing that caused us pain. It was the first cause in a long lineage of causes and effects.

That first cause is like the grain of sand that was introduced into the clam's shell to eventually create the pearl. It is the small center of the snowball that was sent down the hill out of control. We wish we could pull those things back. We wish we could stop the avalanche of events. We wish we knew how or what they even were.

In the worlds of energy, there is no time and space. In energy, you are happy and whole. The goal is to get back to that reality in the present. The way to do that is to reach through time and space with your intention and remove that first domino. You want to eliminate that first cause in the chain of reactions so none of the pain that ensues is ever initiated.

(Say each statement 3 times out loud while CONTINUOUSLY tapping on the top of your head at the crown chakra and say it a fourth time while tapping on your chest at the heart chakra. Say each word deliberately. They are not just words but a vibration that you are initiating to shift energy. Pause after each word. Say it in a commanding but even tone, not as a question. Forgo saying it in a singsong tone or with bravado. Say them all.)

"I want the first cause eliminated that initiated weight gain; in all moments."
"I want the first cause eliminated that initiated lack; in all moments."
"I want the first cause eliminated that initiated disease; in all moments."
"I want the first cause eliminated that initiated weakness; in all moments."
"I want the first cause eliminated that initiated fear; in all moments."
"I want the first cause eliminated that initiated want; in all moments."
"I want the first cause eliminated that initiated greed; in all moments."
"I want the first cause eliminated that initiated unworthiness; in all moments."
"I want the first cause eliminated that initiated depression; in all moments."
"I want the first cause eliminated that initiated sadness; in all moments."
"I want the first cause eliminated that initiated imbalance; in all moments."
"I want the first cause eliminated that initiated physical pain; in all moments."

~ ~ ~ ~ ~

"I want the first cause eliminated that initiated emotional pain; in all moments."

"I want the first cause eliminated that initiated mental torment; in all moments."
"I want the first cause eliminated that initiated a sense of separation; in all moments."
"I want the first cause eliminated that initiated hate; in all moments."
"I want the first cause eliminated that initiated slavery; in all moments."
"I want the first cause eliminated that initiated failure; in all moments."
"I want the first cause eliminated that initiated insecurity; in all moments."
"I want the first cause eliminated that initiated rejection; in all moments."
"I want the first cause eliminated that initiated abandonment; in all moments."
"I want the first cause eliminated that initiated pollution; in all moments."
"I want the first cause eliminated that initiated apathy; in all moments."
"I want the first cause eliminated that initiated denial; in all moments."
"I want the first cause eliminated that initiated wearing masks; in all moments."
"I want the first cause eliminated that initiated having walls; in all moments."
"I want the first cause eliminated that initiated wearing armor; in all moments."
"I want the first cause eliminated that initiated coming out of my center; in all moments."
"I want the first cause eliminated that initiated war; in all moments."

"I want the first cause eliminated that initiated manipulation; in all moments."
"I want the first cause eliminated that initiated death; in all moments."
"I want the first cause eliminated that initiated suffering; in all moments."
"I want the first cause eliminated that initiated any schisms; in all moments."
"I want the first cause eliminated that initiated fragmentation; in all moments."
"I want the first cause eliminated that initiated ugliness; in all moments."
"I want the first cause eliminated that initiated discontent; in all moments."
"I want the first cause eliminated that initiated ignorance; in all moments."
"I want the first cause eliminated that initiated indifference; in all moments."
"I want the first cause eliminated that initiated giving away my power; in all moments."
"I want the first cause eliminated that initiated lack of discernment; in all moments."
"I am centered and empowered in the divinity of wholeness; in all moments."

Doing this exercise may be the best thing you do for yourself.

WEEK 30

The "Doing What You Love" Diet

If you have tried everything to lose weight and nothing works, maybe the fault is in linear dieting. Linear dieting is the belief that every person responds equally to the same experience, every diet is equal for every person and that calories are linear in measurement. I have a theory that all calories are not linear. Meaning that they are not all equal.

Time is not linear. This means that doing something that we love for a minute may feel and be completely different from doing something that we dread for that same minute. If we can screw up something as fundamental as the gauging of time, of course we can screw up most anything else, especially if it has many more variables than time and space.

So what if a calorie is not a linear means of calculation? What if, a calorie of doing what you absolutely love is burned much more quickly than a calorie of doing what you hate. Maybe that is the missing secret for why all those times in the gym don't calculate results. Maybe that is why there are people out there who can eat anything they want and still remain fit. I understand the whole concept of them having brown fat, but what if there is more to it?

~ ~ ~ ~ ~

What if the best diet is simply doing what you love? Fill your day with so much joy and fun that there is a shift in thoughts, feelings and body chemistry. It may be harder to get started because there is so much more resistance. But instead of planning out your whole diet regime, how about using that energy to figure out fun and interesting activities to eat up your time. Get art supplies and use up your down time being creative. When you do physical activity, make certain that it is fun.

The goal is to have as much joy as possible.

~ ~ ~ ~ ~

Also, here is a technique:

What if being loving burned up more calories than stewing in your own juices? Motivate yourself to love everyone to burn calories.

In contemplation, see your heart chakra as this orb in the middle of your chest area. Send out love to the whole world. As you do this, see it getting bigger. Start see it drawing on the energy of the body as a means to give out love to the whole world. See the heart chakra as a huge golden globe in the body getting bigger and bigger as it sends energy out to uplift the whole world. See yourself as an empowered generator of divine love.

Now, see all the fat in your body moving towards the heart chakra and being used to generate all the divine love that you send out to the word. Action follows thought. So convert all your fat cells to energy to send love out to the world. Many of us are overweight because we feel ineffective and powerless. This is a quick and efficient way to drastically change that dynamic.

WEEK 31

The Power of A Pure Intention

The world is run by powerful intentions. It is surprising how few people consciously formulate them. The ones that do are the success stories. When children are little, what intention are they given? Are they taught to use their energies to share their innate talents or change the world? Or are they given the shortsighted intention just to be happy?

Parents want their children to be happy. They are trying to fulfill all that they lacked by showering it on their children. They are using their child for their own therapy in a way. The most consistently dynamic demographic of people are the ones that say they have struggled, and that struggle nurtured a greater intention. These are the ones that succeed: The ones that can hold a pure intention and work towards the manifestation of it.

Why do so many diets fail? The person who is dieting changes the original intention from losing weight, to getting a more shortsighted intention met. If the person is able to hold the original intention through all the body signals that scream for them to change the intention, then they can succeed.

Medicine is an intention. Think about it. When you buy over the counter drugs, you are buying the intention to get rid of your pain. It is a billion dollar industry to give someone an intention in a bottle. It works for so many. I am grateful to have such an intention at my fingertips once in awhile. That is why placebos work. They are infused with the same intention as the real antidote.

It seems that "the intention" is the difference between western and alternative medicine. The intention in western medicine is to patch up the physical body and keep it running at all costs to the quality of life. Its intention is to burn, cut or poison the dis-ease out of the body without ever knowing the root cause.

Alternative medicine's intention is to maintain a quality of life and advocate for wholeness. The body, mind, and spirit are aligned to find the root cause of the disease and to address it in a loving, yet effective way. Instead of rejecting key components of the body because they have been compromised, those parts are still valued. They are even validated more because of the issue. Those parts that are affected with dis-ease are reincorporated back into the whole with a strong and loving intention. Those body parts, similar to the whole individual, are made to feel valued and regain their original intention of helping to run a healthy organism.

~ ~ ~ ~ ~

Somewhere along the way, people lost their drive, spirit or effectiveness. They were made to feel powerless one too many times. SO many left their dignity at the hospital of their insurance company's choosing. Or dropped it out on the floor of a nine to five job. For so many, opting out is actually the only way they feel that they can empower themselves. It is a sad kind of Zen thing of this modern society. The only way to empower oneself is to be ineffective and opt out of society in any of the limited social means possible: disability, welfare, jail, violence or death.

The remedy is to instill strong intentions in our children and ourselves. It is important that everyone understand their own empowerment and claim it back within themselves. Just think about it, if you weren't empowered, the advertising business wouldn't be a trillion dollar industry to woo you. So many people wake up and just accept whatever the day may bring.

Set a strong intention to have a successful day. Do so continuously until you accept the fact that you are creating the success. Choose bigger goals and intentions. Consciously choose to be happy, healthy, wise and free. See how your intentions formulate what you see manifesting around you. Perpetuate this awareness in those you love. Challenge every thought and belief that is diminishing. Ask yourself, "Who benefits from me believing this way?" In this way, you will be sending a ripple of empowerment out that can assist in empowering the whole world. What a great intention!

~ ~ ~ ~ ~

More Taps To Address Food Issues

(Say each statement three times while tapping on your head and say it a fourth time while tapping on your chest.)

"I release eating foods that are bad for me; in all moments."
"I release eating foods that deplete my energy; in all moments."
"I release eating foods that weigh me down; in all moments."
"I release eating foods that cause me to feel more hungry; in all moments."
"I release using foods to plug a void; in all moments."
"I release using food to sop up the sadness; in all moments."
"I release considering going out to eat as an adventure; in all moments."
"I release using food for entertainment; in all moments."
"I release using food to feel normal; in all moments."
"I release craving sugar to feel love; in all moments."
"I release craving fats to feel safe; in all moments."
"I release the fear of experiencing hunger; in all moments."
"I release overreacting to hunger pains; in all moments."
"I release confusing hunger for imminent death; in all moments."
"I sever all connections between food, hunger and trauma of any kind; in all moments."
"I shift my paradigm to feel empowered when hungry; in all moments."

WEEK 32

Technique to tighten the skin: We assume our body knows what we want it to do. Maybe it doesn't. Maybe the signals get crossed somewhere and it needs to be reminded of what we want it to do. When our skin becomes looser with age or weight loss, we may think it is not capable of tightening again. But it is really resilient. Why not try using the intention of a visualization to tighten your own skin? Have you ever been in a group of people who were gathered in a circle? The circle was a little spread out so the facilitator instructs everyone to tighten the circle. Visualize all your skin cells in groups of loose circles all over your body. Simply instruct them all to tighten their circles. Visualize all these little beings joining hands and tightening their bonds. See them go from scattered groups to organized, joyful, cohesive circles. Make it part of your daily routine. See what happens.

~ ~ ~ ~ ~

Instinctual Eating

They are preaching so hard to get us to eat that breakfast. For years, I have been listening to them against my own innate wisdom. Now I realize why my instincts told me *not* to eat breakfast. *Because it is not good for me.*

Eating breakfast interrupts my body's own natural cycle of telling me when I am hungry. It makes me crave that second meal all too soon and keeps my mind on food way more than necessary. If I don't eat first thing in the morning, I am less hungry, I think about food less, and I consume less in a day. I am starting to wonder what came first, people overeating or the "experts" pushing breakfast on everyone.

~ ~ ~ ~ ~

I have been researching brown fat versus white fat. Brown fat is what people who eat all they want and never gain weight have. Brown fat has way more oxygen receptors on it, meaning it burns up energy more quickly. Brown fat *eats* white fat. As we get older, our brown fat reserves dwindle. That may be why, as we age, our metabolism slows down.

Brown fat is associated with longevity. The body keeps making brown fat when there are stints of not eating. To go longer in the day without eating is more conducive to making brown fat. Eating those micro meals just insures that there will be no brown fat production. The people who live the longest are people in countries where food is sometimes scarce and they are forced to fast. That fasting leads to the production of brown fat.

In the 70's, fasting was popular. Most likely, people figured out that it was healthy. It has always bothered me to eat breakfast. But I listened to the experts on every morning show. It has contributed much to overeating in myself. When I was younger and went without eating, I felt empowered. I am starting to realize that wasn't just psychological. It was the physical body being validated.

There is a strength in listening to the body. It aligns the body with the mind and even the emotions. Everything is more expressive when it is listened to, including the intuitive centers of the body. If we listen to our body about when to eat, maybe we will also listen to it about what to eat. This is what I have experienced. Maybe it is not as much about dieting but giving the body a voice on what it wants. Maybe then, the mind and emotions will loosen their grip on the body. Maybe then the body, mind and emotions will all align, and good health and fitness will reign.

We have all been warned about emotional eating. But mental eating is not the answer. Instinctual eating is the key. It is the only one that validates the body. Eating when the body tells us it is time is the only system that supports the validity of the body's importance. By validating the innate wisdom of the physical body, it no longer has to "act out" by creating dis-ease. It also negates the need to make itself bigger to validate it.

If no amount of dieting has worked for you, and you are not under doctor's orders, you may want to try instinctual eating for a change. Maybe it will be surprisingly easy to regulate the body's intake once you let it decide when to eat.

WEEK 33

Taps for Food Confusion

(Say each statement 3 times out loud while tapping on the top of your head at the crown chakra and say it a fourth time while tapping on your chest at the heart chakra)

"I release using food as a form of entertainment; in all moments."
"I release confusing food for entertainment; in all moments."
"I release needing food to feel entertained; in all moments."
"I release being emotionally vested in food; in all moments."
"I release using food to define my happiness; in all moments."
"I release associating food with home and family; in all moments."
"I release associating food with love; in all moments."
"I release associating food with joy; in all moments."
"I release overindulging to feel abundant; in all moments."
"I release eating more to feel more loved; in all moments."

~ ~ ~ ~ ~

"I release eating more to feel happier; in all moments."

"I release eating more to feel a better sense of home and family; in all moments."
"I release being programed to eat more; in all moments."
"I remove all food related engrams; in all moments."
"I shift my paradigm from food to spontaneous Joy, Love, Abundance and a feeling of home and family; in all moments."
"I transcend all food miscues; in all moments."
"I am centered and empowered in being perpetually fed by Joy, Love, Abundance Freedom, Life and Wholeness; in all moments."

~ ~ ~ ~ ~

Others are not thinking about you in a negative way. If they have slighted you or hurt your feelings, they may not even realize it. You are the only one carrying it around most times. So literally drop it and let it go.

WEEK 34

For Everyone Who Struggles With Food Issues: Food Issue Marathon

This is for anyone who has tried every diet and still struggles with food issues. (Say each statement three times while tapping on your head and say it a fourth time while tapping on your chest.)

"I release confusing food for love; in all moments."
"I release confusing food for friendship; in all moments."
"I release confusing food for fun; in all moments."
"I release confusing food for security; in all moments."
"I release confusing food for sex; in all moments."
"I release confusing food for intimacy; in all moments."
"I release confusing food for adventure; in all moments"
"I release confusing food for family; in all moments."
"I release confusing food for confidence; in all moments."
"I release confusing food for a relationship; in all moments."
"I release confusing food for power; in all moments."
"I release confusing food for success; in all moments."
"I release confusing food for love; in all moments."

"I release confusing food for companionship; in all moments."
"I release confusing food for peace; in all moments."
"I release confusing food for likability; in all moments."

"I release confusing food for beauty; in all moments."
"I release being addicted to food; in all moments."
"I release confusing food for family; in all moments."
"I release confusing food for friendship; in all moments."
"I shatter the illusion of food; in all moments."
"I release using food as a crutch; in all moments."

"I release replacing my joy with food; in all moments."
"I release replacing love with food; in all moments."
"I release inhibiting my own creativity by eating food; in all moments."
"I release trading in my abundance for food; in all moments."
"I release choosing food over freedom; in all moments."
"I release confusing food for reality; in all moments."
"I release choosing food over reality; in all moments."
"I release using food as a security blanket; in all moments."
"I release allowing food to dumb down my consciousness; in all moments."
"I release choosing food over adventure; in all moments."
"I release choosing food over life; in all moments."
"I release lowering my vibration with food; in all moments."
"I release being manipulated by food; in all moments."
"I shift my paradigm from food to Joy, Love, Abundance, Freedom, Health, Success, Security, Companionship, Peace, Life, and Wholeness; in all moments."

WEEK 35

"I release the primal need to forage for food; in all moments."
"I release using foraging for food as a distraction from stress; in all moments."
"I release mourning my own innocence; in all moments."
"I release mourning a more innocent time; in all moments."
"I release the trauma of starving to death; in all moments."
"I release confusing hunger with starving to death; in all moments."
"I release the guilt of eating; in all moments."
"I release trying to feed the whole group through my body; in all moments."
"I dry up the void of depravity within; in all moments."
"I dry up the inner hunger; in all moments."
"I release defining being thin as unhealthy; in all moments."
"I release associating being thin with disease and poverty; in all moments."
"I release the trauma of being poor and diseased; in all moments."
"I release associating being thin as being invisible; in all moments."

~ ~ ~ ~ ~

"I release confusing being thin with being weak; in all moments."
"I release the fear of being weak; in all moments."
"I release protecting myself in a big body; in all moments."
"I release using weight to compensate for feeling weak; in all moments."
"I release confusing carrying extra weight with being strong and safe; in all moments."
"I release the fear of being attractive; in all moments."
"I release hiding my beauty; in all moments."
"I release using weight to hide; in all moments."
"I embrace my own beauty; in all moments."
"I release eating out of boredom; in all moments."
"I release eating as a coping mechanism; in all moments."
"I release eating because I am sad; in all moments."
"I release eating to fill a void; in all moments."
"I release eating to feel loved; in all moments."
"I release eating to feel comfort; in all moments."

~ ~ ~ ~ ~

"I release eating to feel safe; in all moments."
"I release eating to kill time; in all moments."
"I release eating to feel busy; in all moments."
"I release eating as a form of distraction; in all moments."
"I release eating for entertainment; in all moments."
"I release eating to be social; in all moments."
"I release eating to celebrate; in all moments."

"I release thinking of food as a friend; in all moments."
"I release the fear of being hungry; in all moments."
"I release eating to nurture myself; in all moments."
"I release being obsessed with food; in all moments."
"I release using food as a hobby; in all moments."
"I am centered and satiated in Joy, Love, Abundance, Freedom, Health, Life and Wholeness; in all moments."

WEEK 36

"I release the fear of being hungry; in all moments."
"I release confusing hunger for death; in all moments."
"I release going into survival mode when I am hungry; in all moments."
"I release defining a huge meal as security; in all moments."
"I release defining a huge meal as love; in all moments."
"I release confusing sugar for love; in all moments."
"I release confusing fatty foods with security; in all moments."
"I release the fear of not having enough; in all moments."
"I release perceiving mealtime as a competition; in all moments."
"I release all the pain and trauma of dying of starvation from my mealtime ritual; in all moments."
"I release confusing dieting with despair; in all moments."
"I release confusing dieting with suicide; in all moments."
"I release storing emotional issues in my physical body; in all moments."
"I release using my body for emotional storage; in all moments."
"I release declaring myself fat; in all moments."
"I release eating shame; in all moments."
"I release protecting myself in fat; in all moments."
"I release insulating myself from pain; in all moments."
"I recant all vows and agreements between myself and fat; in all moments."

"I remove all curses and blessings between myself and fat; in all moments."
"I dissolve all karmic ties between myself and fat; in all moments."
I remove all the pain, burden and limitations that fat has put on me; in all moments."
"I take back all the Joy, Love, Abundance, Freedom, and Wholeness that fat has taken from me; in all moments."
"I release resonating with fat; in all moments."
"I release emanating with fat; in all moments."
"I remove all fat from my sound frequency; in all moments."
"I remove all fat from my light body; in all moments."
I shift my paradigm from fat to Joy, Love, Abundance, Freedom, Health and Wholeness; in all moments."

~ ~ ~ ~ ~

"I release all the issues stored in all fat cells; in all moments."
"I release holding on to fat cells; in all moments."
"I release identifying with fat cells; in all moments."
"I release personifying a fat cell; in all moments."
"I release using fat cells to protect myself; in all moments."
"I release the genetic propensity to rely on fat cells; in all moments."
"I release using fat cells as a buffer; in all moments."
"I release being at the mercy of fat cells; in all moments."

"I release using fat cells for solace; in all moments."
"I release using fat cells to define myself; in all moments."
"I recant all vows and agreements between myself and all fat cells; in all moments."
"I collapse all fat cells; in all moments."
"I remove all curses and blessings between myself and all fat cells; in all moments."
"I dissolve all karmic ties between myself and all fat cells; in all moments."
"I cut all the cords and ties to all fat cells; in all moments."
"I remove all the pain, burden, limitations, and engrams that all fat cells have put on me; in all moments."
"I take back all the joy, love, abundance, freedom, health, success, security, companionship, creativity, peace, life, wholeness, beauty, enthusiasm and adventure that all fat cells have taken from me; in all moments."
"I withdraw all my energy from all fat cells; in all moments."
"I dissolve all fat cells into divine love; in all moments."
"I release harboring fat cells; in all moments."
"I release resonating with fat cells; in all moments."
"I release emanating with fat cells; in all moments."
"I remove all fat cells from my sound frequency; in all moments."
"I remove all fat cells from my light body; in all moments."
"I shift my paradigm from all fat cells to joy, love, abundance, freedom, health, success, security, companionship, creativity, peace, life, wholeness, beauty, enthusiasm and adventure; in all moments."

"I transcend all fat cells; in all moments."
"I am centered and empowered in joy, love, abundance, freedom, health, success, security, companionship, creativity, peace, life, wholeness, beauty, enthusiasm and adventure; in all moments."

~ ~ ~ ~ ~

"I amp up my metabolism; in all moments."
"I encourage my stem cells to create more brown fat; in all moments."
"I regenerate the production of brown fat in my body; in all moments."
"I command the PRDM16 molecules to produce brown fat; in all moments."
"I empower the BMP-7 protein to produce brown fat; in all moments."
"I uptake my body's levels of melatonin; in all moments."
"I make space in this world for the mitochondria of my fat cells to have express levels of UCP1 protein; in all moments."
"I remove all blockages to the mitochondria of my fat cells to have express levels of UCP1 protein; in all moments."
"I stretch the capacity of the mitochondria of my fat cells to have express levels of UCP1 protein; in all moments."
"I make space in my body for more brown fat; in all moments."

"I remove all blockages and limiting beliefs to having more brown fat in my body; in all moments."
"I stretch my body's capacity to manufacture brown fat; in all moments."
"I recalibrate my body to empower the brown fat; in all moments."
"I awaken and empower my body's brown fat to use up all the white fat; in all moments."
"I command my body to use up all the white fat; in all moments."
"I shift my body's paradigm from white fat to brown fat; in all moments."
"I am centered and empowered in brown fat; in all moments."
"I recant all vows and agreements between myself and starvation; in all moments."
"I remove all curses and blessings between myself and starvation; in all moments."
"I dissolve all karmic ties between myself and starvation; in all moments."
I remove all the pain, burden and limitations that starvation has put on me; in all moments."
"I take back all the Joy, Love, Abundance, Freedom, and Wholeness that starvation has taken from me; in all moments."
"I release resonating with starvation; in all moments."
"I release emanating with starvation; in all moments."
"I remove all of starvation from my sound frequency; in all moments."
"I remove all of starvation from my light body; in all moments."

I shift my paradigm from starvation to Joy, Love, Abundance, Freedom, Health and Wholeness; in all moments."
"I recant all vows and agreements between myself and food; in all moments."
"I remove all curses and blessings between myself and food; in all moments."
"I dissolve all karmic ties between myself and food; in all moments."
I remove all the pain, burden and limitations that food has put on me; in all moments."
"I take back all the Joy, Love, Abundance, Freedom, and Wholeness that food has taken from me in all moments."
"I release resonating with food; in all moments."
"I release emanating with food; in all moments."
"I remove all food from my sound frequency; in all moments."
"I remove all food from my light body; in all moments."
I shift my paradigm from food to Joy, Love, Abundance, Freedom, Health and Wholeness; in all moments."

WEEK 37

Taps to Drop Unwanted Weight

(Say each Statement three times while tapping on your head and say it a fourth time while tapping on your chest.)

"I release carrying around thoughts as extra weight on my body; in all moments."
"I release carrying around feelings as extra weight on my body; in all moments."
"I release carrying around memories as extra weight on my body; in all moments."
"I release carrying around traumas as extra weight on my body; in all moments."
"I release carrying around opinions and judgments as extra weight on my body; in all moments."
"I release carrying around jealousies as extra weight on my body; in all moments."
"I release carrying around unworthiness as extra weight on my body; in all moments."
"I release carrying around grudges as extra weight on my body; in all moments."
"I release carrying around regrets as extra weight on my body; in all moments."
"I release carrying around frustrations as extra weight on my body; in all moments."
"I release carrying around past lovers as extra weight on my body; in all moments."
"I release carrying around mistakes as extra weight on my body; in all moments."

"I release carrying around wrong choices as extra weight on my body; in all moments."
"I release carrying fears as extra weight on my body; in all moments."
"I release carrying self-punishment as extra weight on my body; in all moments."
"I release carrying sadness as extra weight on my body; in all moments."
"I release carrying around indoctrination or shame as extra weight on my body; in all moments."

~ ~ ~ ~ ~

"I release engaging in short-term solutions for long-term issues; in all moments."
"I eliminate the first cause in regards to all long-term issues; in all moments."
"I eliminate the first cause in regards to perpetuating long-term issues; in all moments"

~ ~ ~ ~ ~

To Alleviate Cravings:

(say each statement three times while tapping on your head and say it a fourth time while tapping on your chest)

"I infuse savory satisfaction into my Sound Frequency and Light Emanation; in all moments"

"I infuse savory satisfaction into all 32 layers of my auric field; in all moments"
"All of my bodies are immersed in and embody savory satisfaction; in all moments"
"I am centered, empowered and imbued in savory satisfaction; in all moments"
"I resonate, emanate and succeed in all my endeavors in savory satisfaction; in all moments"

WEEK 38

Stop Binge Eating

Foraging for food is a primal behavior. It is ingrained as a survival tool in the makeup of all animals. It is a necessity to survive in the wild. What separates man from the animal kingdom is his lack of need to forage anymore. But this behavior is so ingrained in our DNA.

When we are stressed, we use foraging for food as a means to return to simpler times. That is what we are doing when we obsess over what to eat. We put a lot of energy into "our next kill" which is usually something really heavy in carbs, fat and sugar that will fill us up. This feeling of wanting to be that full is a means of wanting to return to simpler times when we were able to take down a kill and gorge upon it. In those simpler times, being so filled with food was a form of security because we knew we would survive another day.

When we gorge like this in groups, as in big holiday meals, it is a primal urge to return to the pack. In the wild, when everyone has gorged after a kill, it registers as safety and serenity because if there were danger around, the group wouldn't be relaxed and gorging on food. These are all primal associations that are being triggered by planning the perfect meal and binge eating.

~ ~ ~ ~ ~

Here are some taps to interrupt the process of primal foraging and gorging, which may have been unconsciously causing binge eating in this present life.

(Say each statement 3 times while tapping on your head and say it a 4th time while tapping on your chest)

"I release obsessively foraging for food; in all moments."
"I release the primal urge to "take down a kill"; in all moments."
"I release using foraging and gorging to return to simpler times; in all moments."
"I release the genetic propensity to forage for food; in all moments."
"I release stress triggering the primal indicator that I have to forage or gorge; in all moments."
"I release associating binge eating with the proactive activity of foraging; in all moments."
"I release associating binge eating and gorging with productivity; in all moments."

~ ~ ~ ~ ~

"I release associating being gorged with safety and peace; in all moments."
"I remove all vivaxes between stress and foraging for food; in all moments."
"I remove all vivaxes between stress and gorging on food; in all moments."
"I remove all programming and conditioning that foraging and gorging have put on me; in all moments."

"I shift my paradigm from obsessive foraging and gorging to a steady calm of peace, resolve and contentment; in all moments."
"I release rejecting contentment as boredom; in all moments."
"I release confusing binge eating with adventure; in all moments."
"I withdraw all my energy form binge eating and obsessive foraging; in all moments."

WEEK 39

(Two weeks of Marathon Taps)

I release resonating with fat; in all moments.
I release emanating with fat; in all moments.
I remove all fat from my Sound frequency; in all moments.
I remove all fat from my Light body; in all moments.
I shift my paradigm from fat to Joy, Love, Abundance, Freedom, Health, and Wholeness; in all moments.
I release all the issues stored in all fat cell; in all moments.
I release holding on to fat cells; in all moments.
I release identifying with fat cells; in all moments.
I release personifying a fat cell; in all moments.
I release using fat cells to protect myself; in all moments.
I release the genetic propensity to rely on fat cells; in all moments.

~ ~ ~ ~ ~

I release using fat cells as a buffer; in all moments.
I release being at the mercy of fat cells; in all moments.
I release using fat cells for solace; in all moments.
I release using fat cells to define myself; in all moments.
I recant all vows and agreements between myself and all fat cells; in all moments.
I remove all curses and blessings between myself and all fat cells; in all moments.

I dissolve all karmic ties between myself and all fat cells; in all moments.
I cut all the cords and ties to all fat cells; in all moments.
I remove all the pain, burden, limitations, and engrams that all fat cells have put on me; in all moments.
I take back all the joy, love, abundance, freedom, health, success, security, companionship, creativity, peace, life, wholeness, beauty, enthusiasm, and adventure that all fat cells have taken from me; in all moments.

~ ~ ~ ~ ~

I withdraw all my energy from all fat cells; in all moments.
I dissolve all fat cells into divine love; in all moments.
I release harboring fat cells; in all moments.
I release resonating with fat cells; in all moments.
I release emanating with fat cells; in all moments.
I remove all fat cells from my Sound frequency; in all moments.
I remove all fat cells from my Light body; in all moments.
I shift my paradigm from all fat cells to joy, love, abundance, freedom, health, success, security, companionship, creativity, peace, life, wholeness, beauty, enthusiasm, and adventure; in all moments.
I transcend all fat cells; in all moments.
I am centered and empowered in joy, love, abundance, freedom, health, success, security, companionship, creativity, peace, life, wholeness, beauty, enthusiasm, and adventure; in all moments.

WEEK 40

(Marathon Taps Continued)

I amp up my metabolism; in all moments.
I encourage my stem cells to create more brown fat; in all moments.
I regenerate the production of brown fat in my body; in all moments.
I commend the PRDM16 molecules to produce brown fat; in all moments.
I empower the BMP-7 protein to produce brown fat; in all moments.
I uptake my body's levels of melatonin; in all moments.
I make space in this world for the mitochondria of my fat cells to have express levels of UCP1 protein; in all moments.
I remove all blockages to the mitochondria of my fat cells to have express levels of UCP1 protein; in all moments.
I stretch the capacity of the mitochondria of my fat cells to have express levels of UCP1 protein; in all moments.

~ ~ ~ ~ ~

I make space in my body for more brown fat; in all moments.
I remove all blockages and limiting beliefs to having more brown fat in my body; in all moments.
I stretch my body's capacity to manufacture brown fat; in all moments.

I recalibrate my body to empower the brown fat; in all moments.
I awaken and empower my body's brown fat to use up all the excess white fat; in all moments.
I command my body to use up all the excess white fat; in all moments.
I shift my body's paradigm from white fat to brown fat; in all moments.
I am centered and empowered in brown fat; in all moments.
I recant all vows and agreements between myself and starvation; in all moments.
I remove all curses and blessings between myself and starvation; in all moments.
I dissolve all karmic ties between myself and starvation; in all moments.

~ ~ ~ ~ ~

I remove all the pain, burden and limitations that starvation has put on me; in all moments.
I take back all the Joy, Love, Abundance, Freedom, and Wholeness that starvation has taken from me; in all moments.
I release resonating with starvation; in all moments.
I release emanating with starvation; in all moments.
I remove all of starvation from my sound frequency; in all moments.
I remove all of starvation from my light body; in all moments.
I shift my paradigm from starvation to Joy, Love, Abundance, Freedom, Health, and Wholeness; in all moments.

I recant all vows and agreements between myself and food; in all moments.
I remove all curses between myself and food; in all moments.
I dissolve all karmic ties between myself and food; in all moments.
I remove all the pain, burden, and limitations that food has put on me; in all moments.
I take back all the Joy, Love, Abundance, Freedom, and Wholeness that food has taken from me; in all moments.
I release resonating with food; in all moments.
I release emanating with food; in all moments.
I remove all food from my Sound frequency; in all moments.
I remove all food from my Light body; in all moments.
I shift my paradigm from food to Joy, Love, Abundance, Freedom, Health, and Wholeness; in all moments.

WEEK 41

An Overlooked Key to Losing Weight

The reason people who are trying to lose weight are supposed to stay away from meat is not because protein makes you fat. It is because the diet industry is in bed with the Food and Drug Administration and doesn't want to step on their toes by telling it like it is.

The reason that people who are dieting can't lose weight if they eat meat may be because the hormones in that meat are used to fatten up the meat. When someone eats the meat, they are also eating those hormones and may suffer the same effect as the meat itself. Hormone-laden beef and poultry have the same effect of fattening up people as they do on beef and poultry.

As a sidebar, woman who want bigger breasts don't need to dream about implants. There is a good possibility they can enlarge their breasts naturally by eating plenty of chicken breast. It is better to try that than indulge in self-mutilation.

"I extract all foreign, fattening agents from my bodily tissue; in all moments."
"I eliminate all foreign, fattening agents from my body; in all moments."
"I flush my system clean of foreign chemicals and agents; in all moments."
"I streamline all organic hormones to support a slim and healthy structure; in all moments."

"I shift my body out of starvation mode; in all moments."
"I release reverting to starvation mode; in all moments."
"I calibrate all my bodily systems and weight to a healthy slim and fit mode; in all moments."
"I regenerate myself to the healthy and vital activity of a pubescent body; in all moments."

~ ~ ~ ~ ~

Honing the Ho'oponopono Technique

There is a technique that helps people heal from all worldly issues by saying four specific statements to those that have been wronged. The premise is that everything in the world that you are aware of is directly related to you, and if you apologize with these four statements, powerful healing occurs.

I AM SORRY
I LOVE YOU
PLEASE FORGIVE ME
THANK YOU

A very subtle tweak of this technique is to use it this way:

Feel into something that brings you a feeling that is not desirable in the body. Think of how your body feels when you eat the wrong food. Feel how the body feels when you feel unworthy or not good enough. Hone into the thickest part of that feeling. Focus on it like a target.

As you hold your attention on that feeling, speak directly to that feeling. Say these four statements very sincerely to those feelings that you have "pinned down." Feel the energy of the issue untangle as palpable as if you were untying a knot. Because that is exactly what is happening.

~ ~ ~ ~ ~

Technique: If you are agitated when you are trying to sleep, bring up all the images that agitate you. As you conjure up the images, imagine that there is a siphon tube in your *liver*. Visualize it drawing all this oily, disgusting, black energy out of your liver and pouring it into a river of Light where it then dissolves. See if this helps you not only fall asleep, but actually wake up feeling lighter.

WEEK 42

Eating Disorders

A client came to me recently. She was distraught about being told she needed a root canal. She really didn't want to get one. She started to tell me that the issue started when she was younger and she would purge. I immediately felt the pain and shame she was holding.

There are two different energetic experiences happening with eating disorders. When someone purges, there is so much incredible pain inside of them that there is no room for anything else. When someone is purging, they are trying to extract the pain. I have had many clients who have not had eating disorders but still have dreams or inner experiences of throwing up thick ugly tar like substance after their private session. They are purging their own pain.

The other experience with eating disorders is that there is a huge abyss within the person that they are trying to plug up with food. Sometimes they will also use other things to try to plug it up, like drugs, alcohol, shopping, smoking or people. When someone can't be alone with themselves and needs to find something to entertain them, that is sometimes a sign that they are feeding a void.

With this particular client, I got the image of her baby teeth. I was shown that the pain we were releasing for her was stored in her physical body in her first molars.

When I told her this, she confirmed that molestation started when she was three years old. As a baby, she processed the emotional pain of being molested into the physical pain of cutting her first molars. This is how emotional pain and physical pain became tangled and confused within her.

I led her through the following taps. After doing the first one, she felt incredibly lighter. After doing a few of them, she cried out joyful saying that she didn't need a root canal at all. She felt the intense experience lift from her. For her, the thought of having a root canal was triggering the experience of being molested. This is part of what was released in her session.

"I release feeding the pain; in all moments."
"I remove the pain; in all moments."
"I recant all vows and agreements between myself and the pain; in all moments."
"I remove all curses and blessings between myself and the pain; in all moments."
"I dissolve all karmic ties between myself and the pain; in all moments."
"I remove all the shame, burden and limitations that pain has put on me; in all moments."
"I withdraw all my energy from the pain; in all moments."
"I take back all the Joy, Love, Abundance, Freedom, Health, Success, Security, Companionship, Peace, Life and Wholeness that the pain has taken from me; in all moments."

~ ~ ~ ~ ~

"I release resonating with the pain; in all moments."
"I release emanating with the pain; in all moments."
"I remove all the pain from my sound frequency; in all moments."
"I remove all the pain from my light body; in all moments."
"I shift my paradigm from pain to Joy, Love, Abundance, Freedom, Health, Success, Security, Companionship, Peace, Life and Wholeness that the pain has taken from me; in all moments."
"I am centered and empowered in Divine Love in all moments."

If you purge, you are going to want to do these. If you binge or indulge in excesses, you are going to want to go through the whole list a second time and switch out the word "void" for "pain." And if you are really feeling freed up from this exercise, you may want to do it a third time and put the word "shame" where the word "pain" is used.

~ ~ ~ ~ ~

Taps of the Day: Release Self-Loathing

"I release hating myself; in all moments."
"I release blaming myself; in all moments."
"I release feeling unworthy; in all moments."
"I release the belief that I am unworthy; in all moments."

"I release lamenting the past; in all moments."
"I release dreading the future; in all moments."
"I release sabotaging my future; in all moments."
"I release being a masochist; in all moments"
"I release having masochistic tendencies; in all moments."
"I release giving away my power; in all moments."
"I release sending mixed signals to the Universe; in all moments."
"I release refusing my gifts; in all moments."
"I release refusing to be gifted; in all moments."
"I shift my paradigm to take in all the wonderment of living in abundance; in all moments."
"I draw all wonderful things to me and receive them graciously; in all moments."
"I am centered and empowered in accepting all things wonderful; in all moments."

WEEK 43

Technique to Fill in the Void

Whenever someone has a need that is out of balance like a compulsion or addiction, they are tapping into a void that has been created around the energy system of the body. It was created by seepage or accessed through a warped or leaky chakra system.

My mother, way back in the seventies, pointed to a specific spot on her throat one day. She explained that when she smokes, she feels a deep satisfaction at that point in her throat. I have experienced the sensation that she is talking about drinking sugary drinks. It is stimulating the throat chakra.

Since then, I realized that any kind of craving or imbalance is attempting to balance or even plug up leakage from a different chakra of the energy system. Smoking, over-talking or eating are ways of addressing the throat chakra. Being addicted to sex is a way to overcompensate at the root chakra. Obsessing over being in love is dealing with the heart chakra.

~ ~ ~ ~ ~

I followed the energy of a craving in myself the other day. When there is a craving, sometimes, it takes on a life and obsession of its own. I was craving something very heavy and savory to "fill me up." I thought I was physically hungry. I ordered a large sub sandwich. I paid attention as the craving in my throat was satiated, and the sheer volume of the meal hit a chakra in my stomach as well. But after eating the whole sub in one sitting, I was still hungry.

By doing this, I was able to uncover a helpful technique to deal with the cravings that seem to have a life of their own and can create obsessive behavior. I discovered access to the "void" that exists when one is trying to overcompensate with a vice. I have discovered a way to deal with that feeling of being a bottomless pit.

Through our physical component, the intangible part of ourselves is able to access all of existence. But this capability isn't acknowledged in us as a species. So many people who access these realms do it unconsciously. I see people's chakras as controlled openings into the infinite. But if the chakras aren't working properly, then an empty space is created around the body of the person. It is created by them "leaking into infinity" and not knowing what to do with this energy. It feels like an extension of the self.

This creates a stagnant space of lifeless energy between their infinite self and them in their physical body. The physical part of themselves registers this void of energy around them as part of themselves. It tries to make it more physical by filling it with the object of their desire. When we are craving something, we are trying to fill up the space around us that we have created through a "leaky" chakra.

~ ~ ~ ~ ~

Technique:

Visualize your own body as an engine to the Divine. See the chakras as gaskets into the infinite realms of possibility. Go through your own chakras and see which ones are warped and not spinning right. These are the ones leaking the infinite around you and creating a void that you deal with by over-indulgence. See your "engine" with all this useless energy around it. It can seem like space around the body that needs to be packed in, or it can look like a huge sack of energy following behind the body like a lawnmower bag.

With your mind and intention, fix all the leaky chakras. Replace the seal on them and re-form the opening, so it is no longer warped. Go through each chakra and address the health of each chakra with the same detail as a Master mechanic working on a leak in an engine. Make certain every issue is addressed. Make sure every chakra is round, sealed and has a healthy spin on it.

After that is done, you have a healthy access to the infinite without the seepage creating void energy around the body. Imagine the sun as a cotton candy like substance of energy. Visualize being able to pluck out big gobs of energy from the sun and packing it around your body to dry up the seepage and to fill in the void.

As you stuff the energy around the body, notice that stagnant energy fill up with healthy energy. See it return to being part of the healthy background energy of the infinite. Keep doing this until there is no empty space around you. Feel the empowerment that this affords you. Feel the magnetic empowerment of having no abnormal buffer between your energy system and the infinite. Sense yourself returning to being part of the infinite with merely a resilient veneer of energy separating you from it.

Next time you have a strong craving or desire, address the chakra that seems to require attention and go through the whole process of fixing all the chakras and packing in the body with light and love. See how it works to minimize the imbalance. This is a powerful technique to empower yourself. May you access your own strength and omnipotence by using it.

WEEK 44

Eating Issues

There are so many different reasons for issues with food. It is not such a cut and dry issue. So when I do sessions with people, I don't always know what is going to need releasing. Here are some reasons for issues with food:

Foraging for food is primal and instinctual. It manifests as binging in this life.
Being poisoned in a past life.
Starving to death.
Starving while having to serve the privileged.
Being eaten alive.
Storing trauma in your body in fat cells.
Being raped or abused for being beautiful so use weight to hide your beauty.
Trying to feed another version of you through over eating.
Trying to feed a village through what you are eating.
Guilt for getting to eat now.
Feeling unworthy of food.
Having to eat putrid food.
Eating inanimate objects to survive.
Watching an animal you raised and love be killed for food.
Punishing yourself for some atrocity that you feel responsible for.

These are all different scenarios that have played out in sessions that have to do with food issues. That is why the sessions are so dynamic. I can narrow down a topic, but until I tune into the energy of the clients, I can't give them specific information. That is why two sessions will never be the same.

~ ~ ~ ~ ~

Gratitude as an Enzyme

When you eat fruits, nuts and vegetables, go back through the process of thanking everyone involved who brought it to you. Thank the growers, deliverers, grocery workers. And if it is a GMO, you may as well thank the factory workers and technicians who made it. Please don't curse anything that is going into your body.

Send out appreciation to the trees or plants it came from. Send appreciation to the roots, the ground, all the nutrients that accumulated into your meal and the rain that quenched your meal's thirst when it was still growing. And most of all, thank the sun for supplying nutrients and energy to your food.

Since plants absorb energy and our body breaks down the food to get that energy, maybe someday we can cut out the middleman and get our sustenance directly from the energy of the world. Until then, use gratitude as a natural enzyme to digest your food better and to give it that "X" factor that may be missing along the way.

~ ~ ~ ~ ~

Find something positive in every situation. If people are complaining about the weather, respond with a positive quip: "I bet the plants are loving the rain."

Pay attention to your thoughts through the day. Catch yourself saying anything negative and stop yourself.

WEEK 45

The Skinny Bitch technique or Stop Kicking the Dog

So many people who are struggling to lose weight focus on the guilt and shame of the experience of eating. Every time you feel guilt and shame when you are eating, you are eating guilt and shame. So every thing you eat, every spoonful, plateful and chip, pour love into it like it is little soldier doing an incredible job in nurturing you.

That is one thing. Throw out the shame and obsession with what the scale says. Focus on how you feel and what your body needs. Shift the blame and guilt to emotional support for your body because it is doing everything it can to support you. It is teamwork. Your body deserves love and kindness.

~ ~ ~ ~ ~

If you are feeling a certain way in your body, it is because your body is working overtime to protect and nurture you. So tell it that you love it, and then it can feel safe and relaxed in doing its job. Your body hates feeling like the enemy all the time. Look at it this way: your body is even safer and more protective of you than a loyal dog. Please give it some acknowledgement. Shaming yourself is kicking the dog.

~ ~ ~ ~ ~

Instead of focusing on the process of eating, use your energy in a more productive way. Try this visualization to shift your expectations of yourself in a positive way. It may seem silly to try this, but no more than shaming yourself with every bite.

You know those people we have met who are naturally very thin? They are the ones who can eat and eat and never gain an ounce. Pull up the memory of all the individuals you've known with this physiology. They have brown fat instead of white fat. Brown fat metabolizes food very quickly.

In visualization, simply see these people surrounding you in a circle. Have them touching you. Two energy systems that are next to each other exchange energy. Visualize the brown cells from these people feeding into your body and see your own fat cells convert into brown fat cells. They will start to process food in an efficient way and dissolve the excess fat cells.

It may seem silly. But it is insanity that this issue has enslaved so many and interrupted their quality of life.

WEEK 46

Fat Shaming

The truth of the matter is that your outer appearance is so insignificant compared to your inner work. Putting so much emphasis on the outer appearance is another form of societal control. It is another way to make someone feel diminished and unfulfilled. There are infinite reasons why people overeat. One of which is that they have starved to death in past lives. The fear of starvation is registered in their DNA. If it takes a lifetime of overeating to reassure people that the experience is over, then that is what they need to do.

Someone who is overweight is using it at a coping mechanism. To shame them is to take someone who is coping with pain and shove more pain into them. Why is that not considered cruel? It makes a person, who is doing the best that they can and is coping in the only way they know, feel unworthy and undesirable because of it. It is a form of abandonment. It can be just as silly and unwarranted as shaming someone who has come back from war for having post-traumatic stress disorder.

~ ~ ~ ~ ~

Here are just some of the reasons for being over weight or over eating:

- Starving in a past life

- Modern foods are engineered to make you fatter as an illusion to make humans seem fulfilled
- Modern foods are engineered to make you hungrier to sell more products
- Advertisements brainwash people to eat more
- Social situations are centered around indulgence
- Binging can be reverting to a peaceful, primal lifetime of being a gatherer
- Trying to feed an aspect of yourself that starved in a past lifetime
- Guilt over being able to eat when others have starved and trying to feed a whole village indirectly because of this
- Keeping layers of fat on you as a form of protection
- Wanting to be undesirable so you don't get sacrificed for your beauty
- Wanting to be undesirable because you have been raped and abused in past times.
- A form of hiding in plain sight
- Associating sugar with love
- Associating fat with security
- Associating eating with a bonding of your people. (In past times people ate big feasts when they were not at war and safe to do so.)
- Grounding your energy so that you feel like you aren't floating away
- Feeling heavy as a way to feel like you do indeed exist and are not invisible
- A way to empower yourself by making your energy big so no one can hurt you
- Fear of not existing

- Memories of eating with a group and trying to reconnect to that experience
- A way to store issues into yourself because you don't want to hurt someone else
- People realizing that it may be their last lifetime to eat food, so they are taking in as much of the experience as possible

These are some of the reasons. There is nothing here about being disgusting or greedy or not caring about oneself. The issue of eating and weight is a very painful experience for the individual. Shaming them is jamming more pain into them. Shaming them is a form of ignorance.

~ ~ ~ ~ ~

In past times, people worked so hard that they needed foods to be hearty. In modern times food has taking on the roll of entertainment. To some of us, it would be easier if we could quit eating altogether like other vices. But food is a primal need like water and air.

Perhaps we can evolve as a species to be able to ingest energy directly from source and not need to eat food at all. Until that happens, just please be kind to others. Just because you can see they are struggling with something, doesn't mean that it is more than someone else is dealing with. It just means that their struggle is more obvious. To kick someone when they are struggling is ignorance at it's best.

Here are some taps to help:

"All algorithms of overeating are dismantled; in all moments."
"All algorithms of weight issues are dismantled; in all moments."

WEEK 47

Release Food Issues

(Say each statement three times out loud while CONTINUOUSLY tapping on the top of your head at the crown chakra and a fourth time tapping on your chest.)

"I release hiding food; in all moments."
"I release being ashamed to eat in front of others; in all moments."
"I release being punished for stealing food; in all moments."
"I release being imprisoned for stealing food; in all moments."
"I release being put to death for stealing food; in all moments."
"I release being ridiculed in regards to food; in all moments."
"I release being forced to serve others food while starving; in all moments."
"I release hating people for eating in front of me; in all moments."
"I release defining going hungry as having integrity; in all moments."
"I release confusing eating as being gluttonous; in all moments."
"I release confusing eating as abusing power; in all moments."
"I release separating myself from those that eat; in all moments."

"I release defining abstaining from food as being spiritual; in all moments."
"I untangle all the confusion in regards to food, eating, morality and my own worth; in all moments."
"I shift my paradigm from fixating on food issues to nurturing myself with Joy, Love, Abundance, Freedom, and Wholeness; in all moments."
"I am centered and empowered in nurturing myself in multifaceted ways; in all moments."
"I satiate myself in Joy, Love, Abundance, Freedom and Wholeness exponentially; in all moments."

~ ~ ~ ~ ~

Eat When You Are Happy!

When you are angry, sad, having feelings of unworthiness or inferiority in any way, you should NEVER eat or drink anything. When you are those things, there are issues releasing from your beingness. It is an energy flow of stagnant issues streaming away from you or being stirred up. These things are best released in as detached a way as possible.

It is good *not* to say, "I am angry or sad," but to say, **"I am releasing anger,** or **"sadness is passing through."** When you identify it that way, you are detaching from it and allowing it to leave instead of melding it with your sense of self.

When you are feeling these things and you are eating, you are masticating the feelings into your food and ingesting them as you swallow. You now have them mixed with the meal and coming back into your body in a different form. What you were just willing to release a few minutes ago, you now have to reincorporate into yourself along with the course material of food. It mostly gets stored as a fat cell or plaque and tarter in your body, and you are now wearing it as a reminder of the anger or any other base energy.

~ ~ ~ ~ ~

It is best to unwind and relax before eating a meal. Don't talk about upsetting issues during the meal, and don't argue either. Mealtime should be a neutral, peaceful time if you want to encourage health in your family. Some people, who are so angry that they are uncomfortable in their skin, got this way by not harboring a peaceful setting during mealtime. This is also why it isn't good to eat on the run. As you do this, you are eating your own impatience.

Be loving to yourself by creating a safe loving atmosphere as you eat. It is more important than you realize. It may be the missing component to a healthy diet regime.

WEEK 48

Body Gratitude

Can you change how you think about your body? Instead of judging it on aesthetics, can you just admire it for the incredible journey that you are on together? Can you thank it for its strength and resilience? Can you be in its corner the way that it has been in yours? No one has been more devoted to you than your own body. Can you just appreciate the fact that you have one and you get to be here in this physical world because of it?

Who cares if each hair is in place? Each hair is a receptor for the sensitivities that you have accrued. Who cares if the padding shifts position? It cares about your comfort and safety, not about winning a prize of any kind. Who cares if you don't stand out because of what you look like? Maybe that was the divine plan all along. Everything that a dear friend has ever done for you, your own body has done and more. It has cried for you, laughed with you and left a trail of memories on its terrain as homage to the journey.

Perhaps the physical pain that you feel is the dejection that your body feels. Perhaps if you shift into gratitude for every muscle fiber, bone and corpuscle, your whole health will shift. Stop treating your own body like an indentured servant and start respecting it for the marvel that it is.

Yet More Food Releases

You know all those commercials that we sit through? Their whole purpose is to connect a positive experience with their product so you buy it. All those cravings, all those extra snacks, all those new favorite "must haves" are programmed into you. Here is the cure. These taps will help to undo the programming.

"I release confusing food for love; in all moments."
"I release confusing food for friendship; in all moments."
"I release confusing food for fun; in all moments."
"I release confusing food for security; in all moments."
"I release confusing food for sex; in all moments."
"I release confusing food for intimacy; in all moments."
"I release confusing food for adventure; in all moments."
"I release confusing food for family; in all moments."

~ ~ ~ ~ ~

"I release confusing food for confidence; in all moments."
"I release confusing food for a relationship; in all moments."
"I release confusing food for power; in all moments."
"I release confusing food for success; in all moments."
"I release confusing food for love; in all moments."
"I release confusing food for companionship; in all moments."

"I release confusing food for peace; in all moments."
"I release confusing food for likability; in all moments."
"I release confusing food for beauty; in all moments."

After doing these, you can trade out the word food and replace it with alcohol, beer, shopping, shoes or what whatever your Achilles heal is.

WEEK 49

Food Taps

"I release using food to relate to others; in all moments."
"I release using food as an emotional connection to life; in all moments."
"I release using food as a social outlet; in all moments."
"I release using food as a means to feel plugged in to society; in all moments."

~ ~ ~ ~ ~

"I release needing to eat to have fun; in all moments."
"I release using food to ground; in all moments."
"I release using food to self-medicate; in all moments."
"I release using food as a distraction; in all moments."

~ ~ ~ ~ ~

Technique to Zap the Cravings

Did you ever see someone eating and get disgusted? You are seeing the energetic influences that are enjoying themselves through their meal. Did you ever feel disgusted at yourself when you eat? You are disgusted with these energetic parasites that are feeding as you eat. You didn't think you were disgusted with yourself all this time, did you? It is these energies that cause one to crave.

Use the craving to draw out the energies and as they are feeding, zap them with incredible Light and Love and dissipate them. The next time you eat those sweets that you crave, try it. Think of the meal as the bait and you as one big bug zapper. As you eat the meal, notice how you are feeling. When you identify a loathing feeling, zap it with your higher intention of dissipating it. You will have just killed the energetic parasite. Keep mindful of identifying the feelings and zapping them out. Try it. It is empowering. It doesn't take much to see a shift in your own cravings. All that will be left is the full feeling and the empowerment.

This works with anything out of balance. Anything that we overindulge in can be bait to zap these energies. Any addiction, or impulsive act can be zapped away with this technique. It is very freeing. Try it!

WEEK 50

Taps on Food Issues in Relationship to Male Energy

"I release being less validated than men; in all moments."
"I release being overlooked in lieu of men; in all moments."
"I release being undervalued more than men; in all moments."
"I release being energetically paid less than men; in all moments."
"I release carrying more weight than men; in all moments."
"I release taking on issues more than men; in all moments."
"I release allowing emotional issues to collect upon my body as weight; in all moments."

~ ~ ~ ~ ~

"I release being affected by male energy's indifference; in all moments."
I release packing on the emotional issues; in all moments."
I release the need to make myself bigger to feel like I exist; in all moments."
"I release using my personal size as emotional blackmail to male energy; in all moments."
"I release using physical weight to measure up to male

energy; in all moments."
"I concentrate my effectiveness in a compact healthy body; in all moments."
"I release making myself sick, angry or unhealthy over male energy; in all moments."

~ ~ ~ ~ ~

"I release caring so much about my dynamics with male energy; in all moments."
"I release basing my worth of existence through my correlation with male energy; in all moments."
"I release deferring to male energy; in all moments."
"I release caring if male energy is attracted to me; in all moments."
"I am centered and empowered in my own physical charge of attractiveness and beauty; in all moments."

WEEK 51

MORE taps to Address Food Issues

"I release the fear and trauma of feeling hunger pains; in all moments."
"I remove all engrams that support hunger pains leading to starvation; in all moments."
"I send all energy matrices into the Light and Sound that cause me to overeat; in all moments."
"I command all complex energy matrices that cause me to overeat to be escorted into the Light and Sound by my guides; in all moments."
"I send all energy matrices into the Light and Sound that cause me to crave food; in all moments."
"I command all complex energy matrices that cause me to crave food to be escorted into the Light and Sound by my guides; in all moments."
"I send all energy matrices into the Light and Sound that cause me to crave sugar; in all moments."
"I command all complex energy matrices that cause me to crave sugar to be escorted into the Light and Sound by my guides; in all moments."

~ ~ ~ ~ ~

"I send all energy matrices into the Light and Sound that cause me to crave fats; in all moments."
"I command all complex energy matrices that cause me to crave fats to be escorted into the Light and Sound by my guides; in all moments."

"I send all energy matrices into the Light and Sound that cause me to fear starving; in all moments."
"I command all complex energy matrices that cause me to fear starving to be escorted into the Light and Sound by my guides; in all moments."
"I send all energy matrices into the Light and Sound that cause me to overeat for any reason; in all moments."
"I command all complex energy matrices that cause me to overeat for any reason to be escorted into the Light and Sound by my guides; in all moments."

~ ~ ~ ~ ~

"I send all energy matrices into the Light and Sound that cause me to have an aversion to physical activity; in all moments."
"I command all complex energy matrices that cause me to have an aversion to physical activity to be escorted into the Light and Sound by my guides; in all moments."
"I send all energy matrices into the Light and Sound that cause me to associate being thin with a looming death; in all moments."
"I command all complex energy matrices that cause me to associate being thin with a looming death to be escorted into the Light and Sound by my guides; in all moments."
"I send all energy matrices into the Light and Sound that cause me to fear being attractive; in all moments."
"I command all complex energy matrices that cause me to fear being attractive to be escorted into the Light and Sound by my guides; in all moments."

WEEK 52

How to Dry Up the Hell of Dieting

Last night I was shown the true nature of Hell. It is not really a place of stagnated consciousness. Sure those with a similar state of consciousness may gather together. This is the nature of the spiritual law of vibrations. It means that things that resonate at a similar sound frequency gravitate to others of the same frequency.

That means that when your family is nasty to you and you can't understand why, it is simply the spiritual law of vibrations coming into play. It doesn't mean that you are not worthy of kindness. Perhaps they are not capable of registering your kindness. Perhaps your kindness is like a high-pitched sound to them that only dogs can hear.

The spiritual laws are as exacting as the law of gravity. So they really aren't anything to take personally. In the other realms last night, my sister and I were driving to look at this property that they were giving away to anyone who could settle in it. It was difficult to locate and that was part of why it was hard to find.

The land itself was next to an expansive ocean, which is symbolic for the God state that everyone wishes to attain. That is how beautiful and pristine this property was. But as you got off the parkway to ride along the oceanfront, there was a long strip of land where the energies were beckoning the drivers to join them.

The energies were vile and performing acts of debauchery. They were dark and hideous exploiting all aspects of themselves to get passersby to join them. Yes, some would be terrified of it, but we are savvy travelers and knew enough to just keep driving. But yes, others would get snared here.

But what was unusual about the area is that it was dwindling in area. In fact, the reason that the prime real estate was being doled out was to dry up this area of the beach. It was a huge area, and it was an eyesore and a problem. Those who had a very different vibratory rate than the ones in the debauchery zones were being given homes nearby to change the vibration of the hell zone.

People think hell is a fixed place. It is a vibration. A state of consciousness. At one point, we drove past the entrance of the park-like setting we were looking for and had to drive by the hell zone again. The first time it was very intimidating. But the second time, I noticed one or two of the images had the same exact movement. They were not as real as I thought they were. They were similar to film screen images. They were similar to habitual behavior. Isn't that all habitual behavior is? There is no consciousness in it.

When I awoke, I realized that the new homes were being offered to anyone who transcended. They are taking up residency right near the boundaries of pure heaven. From there, they are able to travel all the worlds and have a ship upon the seas of God as well. Their function will be to dry up those places of lower vibration simply by existing as they do and maintaining their own integrity. Isn't that what we all do here?

I realized the one core issue of all those who were in hell. It was not an issue of worthiness. No one is worthy of hell. Or, more accurately, no one is unworthy of heaven. We are all offshoots of love individualizing the experience of love and reporting back to Source as a means to expand the borders of love. If one is experiencing hellish things, it just makes the move sweeter and more greatly appreciated when they return to balance.

No one is bad or evil. No. The one defining issue that collected the abominations that I saw in one place was regret. Regret was the heavy vibration that attracted more of the same. If gratitude is associated with wonderful things, regret is its antonym. See, hell isn't a place but a state of consciousness. It is being stuck in a ditch that seems too steep to get out of. Have you ever met someone stuck in regret? They are entrenched. Regret needs to be addressed with as much gratitude as possible to keep out of the negative trenches.

It is subtle. *Why doesn't anyone like me? Why wasn't I born beautiful, popular, or with loving parents? Why do they love them and not me? Why doesn't my family appreciate me Why did I have that one life-changing incident? Why can't I lose weight? Why can't I just win the lottery?* Understanding this concept IS winning the lottery. You are now capable of moving away from regret and drying up hell by your shift in awareness.

By the way, no hell is private. You subject everyone else to your vibration and add to a disgusting subtle reality when you immerse yourself in regret. When you immerse yourself in regret, you add to hell. Hell, like heaven, doesn't exist in a remote place. It is a vibration that all access through you. You can be a doorway to heaven, hell or both for all others. You choose. You choose, and in their relationship with you, they choose as well.

Have no regrets. Follow your inner promptings. Let love, kindness, awareness, integrity and adventure be your compass. They will keep you out of hell.

Testimonials for *The Do What You Love Diet*

"It seems like my entire life has been lived on a diet. As a teenager there was a doctor-assisted diet where I was given pills for energy, for sleep, for a laxative, for water retention, etc. That was probably the first attempt to control the weight. I could lose some pounds, but for a little while and I would gain it right back, plus extra pounds. Nothing allowed me to keep the weight off. Not the low carb diet, the cabbage soup diet, the liquid diet, or any other diet. I just couldn't do it. It left me feeling frustrated, feeling like a failure and fat. Then five years ago, I connected with Jen and started doing the taps that she offered. I did the taps religiously everyday. I still do. A little over a year ago, Jen started putting out taps for weight control.

"Those taps and all the techniques and visualization were the saving grace for me. Those taps freed me of all the reasons for eating indiscriminately. I don't eat because of any emotion that is being triggered. I eat normal. Now, in little over a year, I have lost sixty-four pounds to date and am keeping the weight off. It seems like the most normal thing in the world. I am not a youth anymore. I eat healthy, enjoy treats when I wish, and don't concern myself with worry of gaining weight again. I am happy, healthy and a size six for the first time in my life. I owe my success to Jen. Not only with the diet taps but with all she so graciously offers. Thank you Jen I. I couldn't have done it without you."

M. M., New York

"After graduating from college, I enlisted in the Marine Corps. I was in the best physical shape of my life. After being discharged and re-entering civilian life, I began to gain weight. One pound a year became 15 pounds extra weight by the time I was in my 40s. After reading Jen's insights and doing the taps and techniques for a year, I am not only my Marine Corps weight but also back in shape. It wasn't that hard either. Thank you Jen."

M.K., Florida

"I have known Jen for over two years. In that time, I've been doing her taps regularly, participating in her group sessions and had private sessions. I never thought that I would lose weight. I wasn't that overweight. I had the belief that *nobody my age who had carried this extra weight for so long needed to or even could lose it*. After a year or so of doing the taps, I lost the extra 10 pounds that I'd had since college. I discovered habitual thoughts and patterns in my eating that only Jen could have helped me break. I discovered I ate negative emotions such as shame and that my eating was connected to past lives. I found the root cause of why I was afraid of being hungry. By doing the taps and the techniques she offered, I released so many negative patterns. It Was NOT about discipline! I am a disciplined person in other aspects of my life. It was about having compassion for myself, becoming more aware, and loving myself. It was about releasing fears I didn't know I had.

"Now, Jen has compiled all these diet, health and awareness taps into this one book to help people with their weight. It is the best non-diet diet. Thank you Jen! Now I feel like I am not afraid with food. It's not about having control, and the fears are gone. Do these taps. Even the ones you think you don't need. They could be the keys to unlock the weight issue. Read and practice the techniques. They work!! And I feel like I've tried everything."

T. A. K. Florida

About The Author

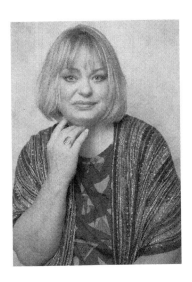

Jen Ward, LMT, is a Reiki Master, an intuitive and gifted healer, and an innovator of healing practices. She is at the leading edge of energy work, providing a loving segue for her techniques to clients, enabling them to cross the bridge of self-discovery with her. Her passion is to empower individuals in their own healing journey, so they can remain in their center every step of the way.

While attending the Onondaga School of Therapeutic Massage, she was first introduced to energy work. It soon became second nature for her to help identify and remove energy blocks from clients. She is highly proficient at tuning into individuals' specific needs to release their issues, allowing their own body to make the energetic changes necessary to return to a greater sense of ease. Her ability to pick up many different modalities as second nature is another aspect of her profound gifts.

Jen is considered a sangoma, a traditional African Shaman, who channels ancestors, emoting sounds and vocalizations in ceremonies. An interesting prerequisite to being a sangoma is to have survived the brink of death. When Jen was first approached with the knowledge of being a sangoma, she had not yet fulfilled this prerequisite. However, in April 2008, when she came back to society on the brink of starvation as a result of traumatic involuntary imprisonment, the qualification had been met. She returned to the world of humanity a devout soul inspired to serve.

Her special abilities have also allowed her to innovate a revolutionary technique for finding lost pets by performing an emotional release on the animal. Using this method, she has successfully reunited many lost pets with their owners.
Jen currently works as a long-distance emotional release facilitator, public speaker, and consultant. Her special modality encompasses a holistic overview of her clients from all vantage points,

including their physical, emotional, causal, and mental areas, ultimately benefiting their work, home, family, and especially spiritual lives.

You can find her work at www.jenuinehealing.com/ or join her Facebook page "Jenuine Healing" at https://www.facebook.com/jenuinehealing.

Jen's Books:

Enlightenment Unveiled: Expound into Empowerment
This book contains case studies to help you peel away the layers to your own empowerment using the tapping technique.

Grow Where You Are Planted: Quotes for an Enlightened "Jeneration"
Inspirational quotes that are seeds to shift your consciousness into greater awareness.

Perpetual Calendar: Daily Exercises to Maintain Balance and Harmony in Your Health, Relationships and the Entire World
369 days of powerful taps to use as a daily grounding practice for those who find meditation difficult.

Children of the Universe
Passionate prose to lead the reader lovingly into expanded consciousness.

Letters of Accord: Assigning Words to Unspoken Truth
Truths that the Ancient Ones want you to know to redirect your life and humanity back into empowerment.

The Do What You Love Diet: Finally, Finally, Finally Feel Good in Your Own Skin
Revolutionary approach to regaining fitness by tackling primal imbalances in relationship to food.

Emerging From the Mist: *Awakening the Balance of Female Empowerment in the World*
Release all the issues that prevent someone from embracing their female empowerment.

Affinity for All Life: *Valuing Your Relationship with All Species*
This book is a means to strengthen and affirm your relationship with the animal kingdom

Made in the USA
San Bernardino, CA
23 September 2017